THE YOGA MANUAL

THE YOGA MANUAL

A Step-by-Step Guide to Gentle Stretching & Total Relaxation

ROSEMARY LESSER

with special photography by
Garth Blore

TODTRI

This book was designed and published by TODTRI Book Publishers

254 West 31st Street, New York, NY 10001-2813

Fax: (212) 695-6984 E-mail: info@todtri.com

Visit us on the web!

www.todtri.com

Printed and bound in Singapore

ISBN 1-57717-093-8

Author: Rosemary Lesser

Publisher: Robert M. Tod
Art Director: Ron Pickless
Editor: Nicolas Wright
Typeset and DTP: Blanc Verso/UK

CONTENTS

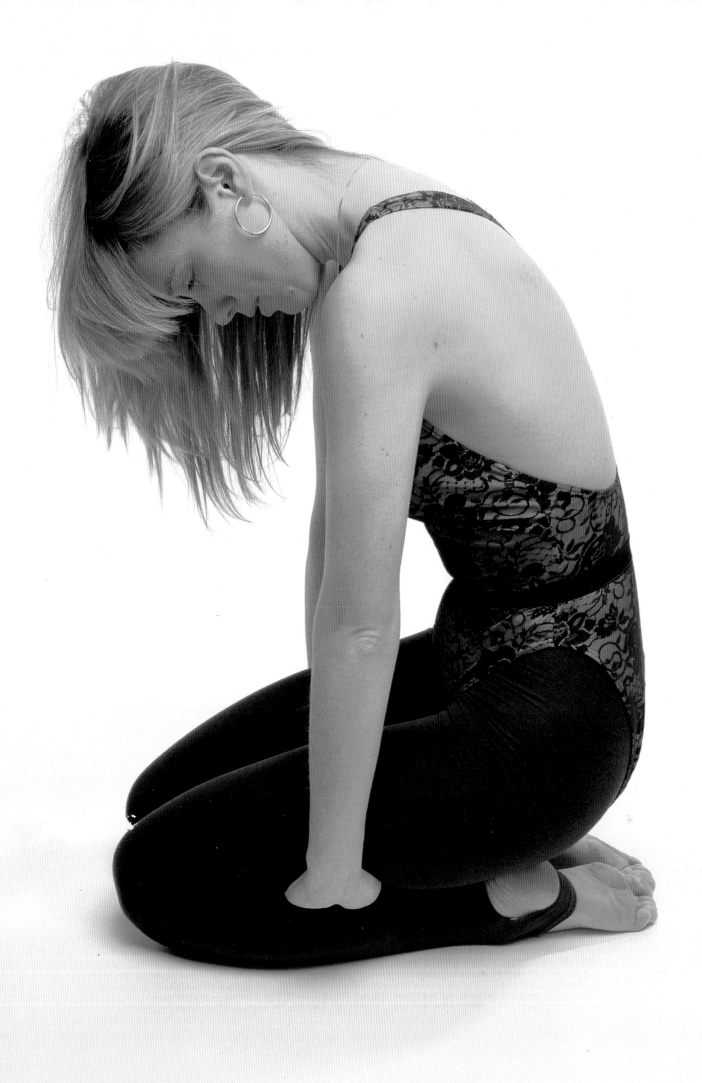

INTRODUCTION

In truth there is nothing new in this book. It is difficult to find anything new to say of Yoga—a way of life thousands of years old. What it aims to do, however, is to present Yoga to those who are new to it in a particularly accessible way.

Yoga can be said to be a philosophy which includes physical and mental disciplines to improve health and vitality. The word is Sanskrit and means Yoke, so we are harnessing ourselves to a particular way of life, but also by its very nature a yoke must be balanced. What we shall experience from Yoga, then, is a balance and union of body, mind and spirit; an equilibrium as we learn to control body, breath and senses. Indeed the Hatha (pronounced Hata) Yoga with which we are concerned in this book is the Yoga usually practiced in the West, a combination of movement, breath control, relaxation and meditation.

Yoga teaches kindness and non-violence, not just to others but to ourselves, and as we benefit so will those with whom we come into contact—the effect of ripples on a pond of love.

Before You Begin

Always remember, **Yoga is individual and non-competitive**. Your own stretch is good enough for you. Listen to your body, it will tell you what feels right at any particular time.

Strive but do not strain in Yoga—if the breath is labored or there is any real discomfort, the stretch has been taken too far—never allow the ego to run ahead of the ability. Everything must be measured by your own comfort.

This book is divided into several chapters with each section making up a Yoga session in itself. **It is advisable to do the postures in the order shown** as this way they are safe and each movement leads the body to a main posture.

Each chapter becomes a little harder than the last, so **don't be in too much of a rush to move on**. Indeed, it is advisable to consult a doctor before beginning Yoga if you have any doubts about your physical condition, or if you are pregnant.

Allow yourself time for Yoga: always begin and end with a period of relaxation to separate yourself from the happenings of life. Work slowly, with awareness and concentration—relax in the postures, reflect after them and relax between them.

Be aware of the device of compensation used in Yoga— your body will often tell you what it wants to do next.

Take care to comply with the guidance on breathing— **breath is life-force and energy**, it is all important.

Before beginning any posture, exhale and tone the lower abdominal muscles—keep control of them throughout.

Find a warm, comfortable place where there is little likelihood of disturbance, and use something as a mat that you will become familiar with and associate with Yoga. Work by candlelight or soft lamp, perhaps play some appropriate soft music.

Wear non-restrictive comfortable clothes and wait at least ninety minutes after a meal before you begin. Whenever possible, close your eyes while practicing Yoga. Nothing you look at is as important as the contemplation of your physical and mental sensations. The Sanskrit names of postures are given of respect for ancient tradition—you don't need to remember them!

Have fun with Yoga—humor keeps the ego in place! Most important of all, enjoy! You deserve it!!

Pranayama and the Chakras

As we breathe we absorb prana, or cosmic energy and life-force, and the practitioner of Yoga will learn to control that energy.

In Yoga, we see an invisible body parallel to our physical one which has nadis or channels running down either side of the spine, and having their upper ends at the opening of the nostrils. The chakras, as we call the centers to which the prana is directed, are placed in strategic positions down the spine.

The channels running down the spine from the nostrils balance the body as they take the prana down the spine: this is because we see the channel from the left nostril,

called ida (symbolizing the moon and our cool, feminine nature) and that from the right nostril called pingala (symbolizing the sun and our warm, masculine temperament), criss-crossing on their way, so balancing the intuitive and aggressive sides of us.

At the same time the chakras are positioned to encourage the activation of important endocrine glands. These glands are the body's natural balancers and our thoughtful and controlled Yoga breathing will stimulate their action. So it is necessary to ensure a straight back when practicing Yoga breathing—only then will there be an uninterrupted flow of breath. We see the chakras associated with the colors of the rainbow.

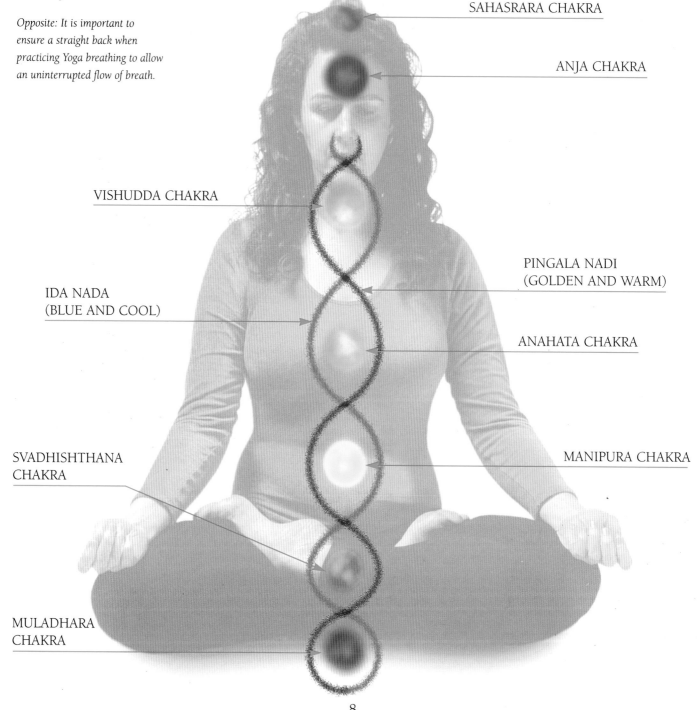

Opposite: It is important to ensure a straight back when practicing Yoga breathing to allow an uninterrupted flow of breath.

SAHASRARA CHAKRA

ANJA CHAKRA

VISHUDDA CHAKRA

PINGALA NADI
(GOLDEN AND WARM)

IDA NADA
(BLUE AND COOL)

ANAHATA CHAKRA

SVADHISHTHANA
CHAKRA

MANIPURA CHAKRA

MULADHARA
CHAKRA

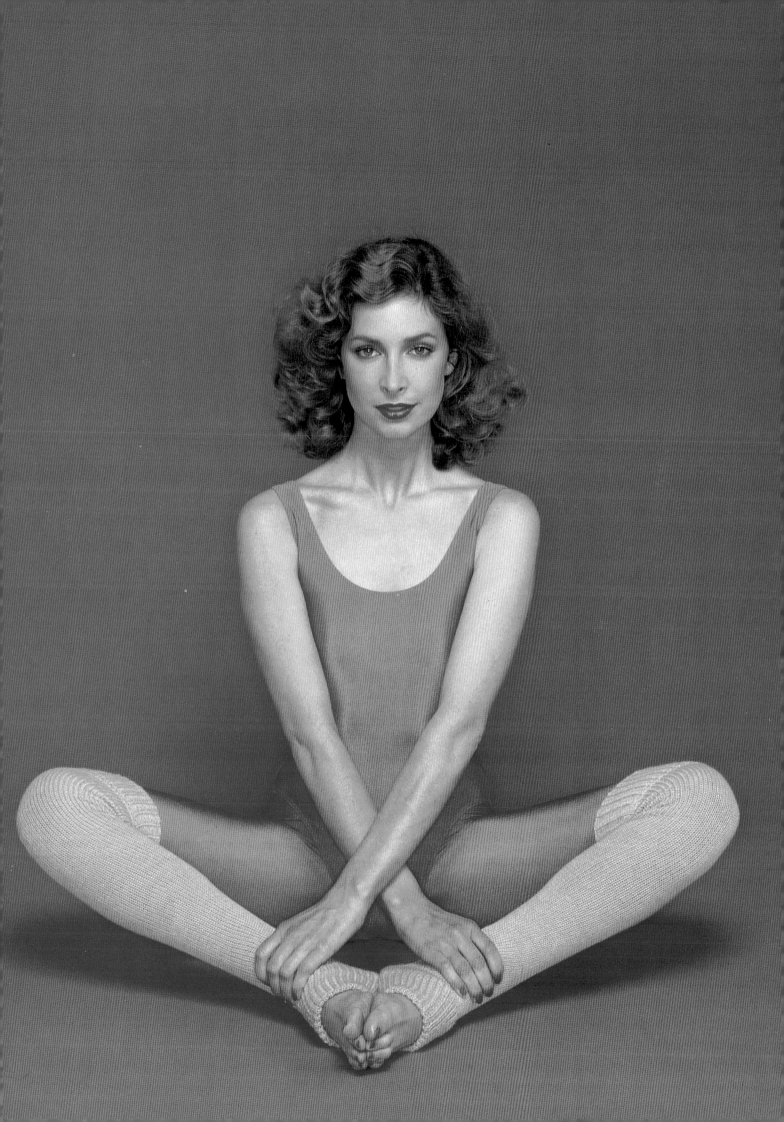

CHAPTER ONE

A FLEXIBLE SPINE

There is a saying in Yoga that you are as old as your spine, and as we begin we will discover a new flexibility in the whole length of the spine and across the shoulders.

Just for today I will try to live through this day only and not tackle my whole life problem at once.

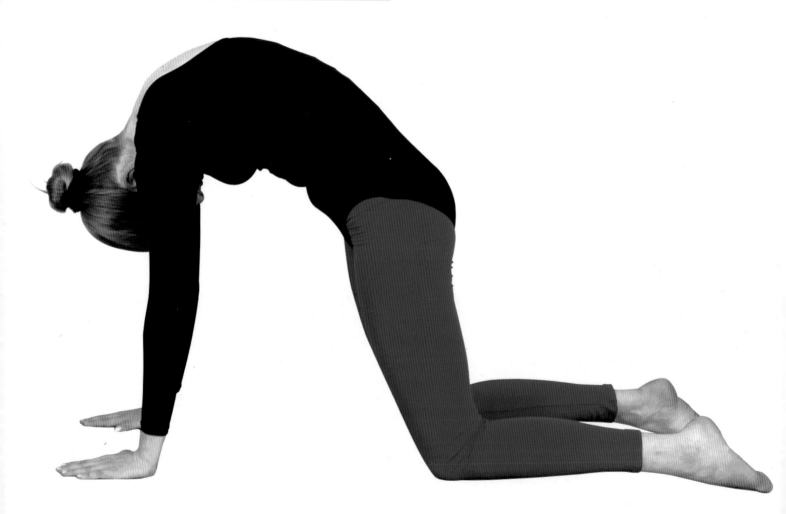

Savasana: "Corpse" Relaxation Posture

Take advantage of the floor beneath you: You can't fall off, so you can really let go. Allow yourself to relax into the floor. Feel your breath become calm, your thoughts begin to slow down. Leave worldly thoughts—those not relevant to your Yoga now—aside.

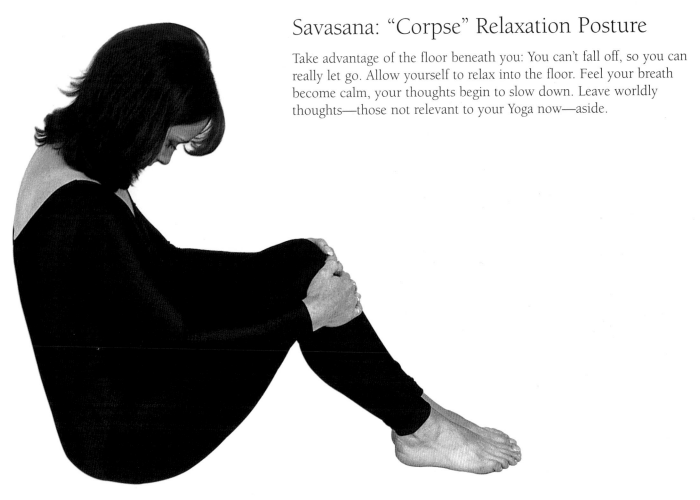

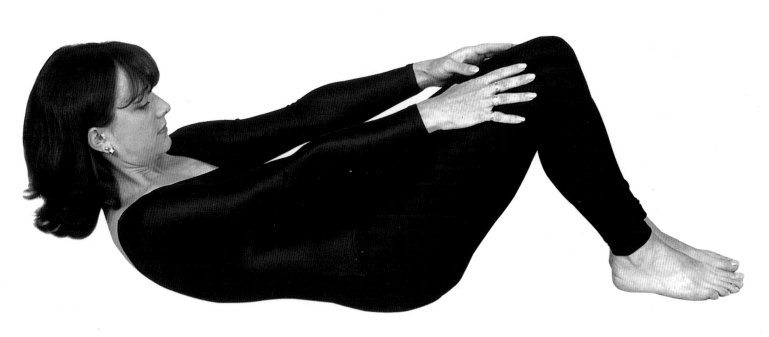

1. Roll the spine down to the mat keeping the chin tucked in and the back of the neck long.

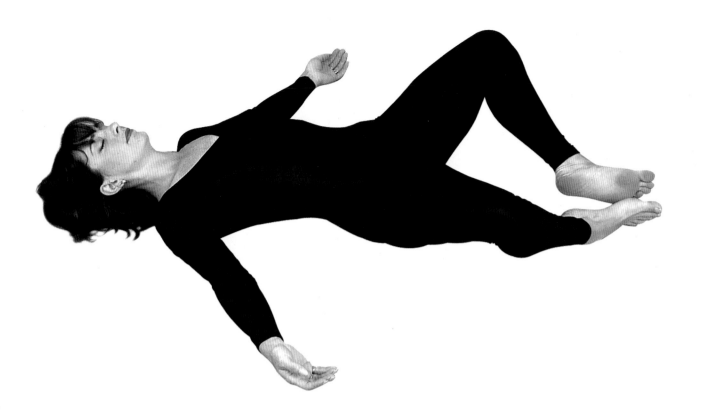

2. Let the knees fall apart and allow the legs to spread and arms fall out to the sides, palms uppermost. If the small of the back is not comfortable, then crook the knees — the back may soon be happy to let them slide away.

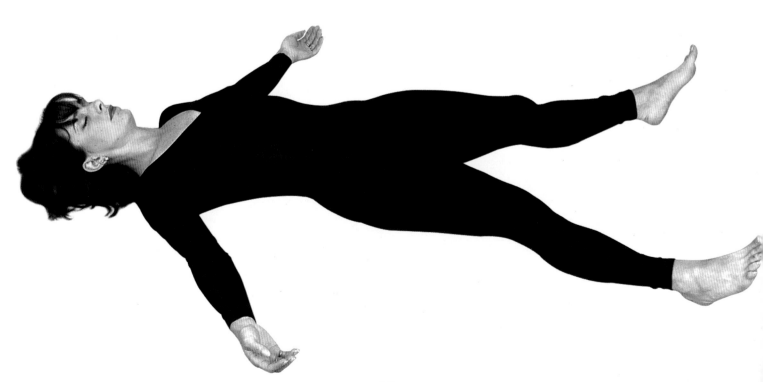

Yastikasana: Stretch

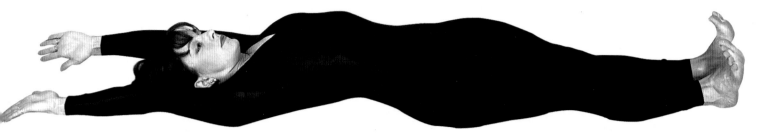

When you are ready, take a long, sensual stretch from heels to fingertips. Yawn.

Grant yourself a moment of peace and you will understand how foolishly you have scurried about.

Learn to be silent and you will notice you have talked too much.

Be kind, and you will realize your judgment of others, and perhaps of yourself, was too severe.

Apanasana: Curl

Bring knees onto chest and hug in for a compensatory curl. Be sure to have exhaled completely if you choose to lift your face towards your knees.

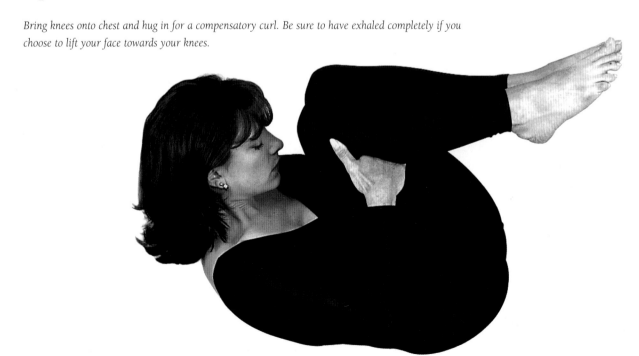

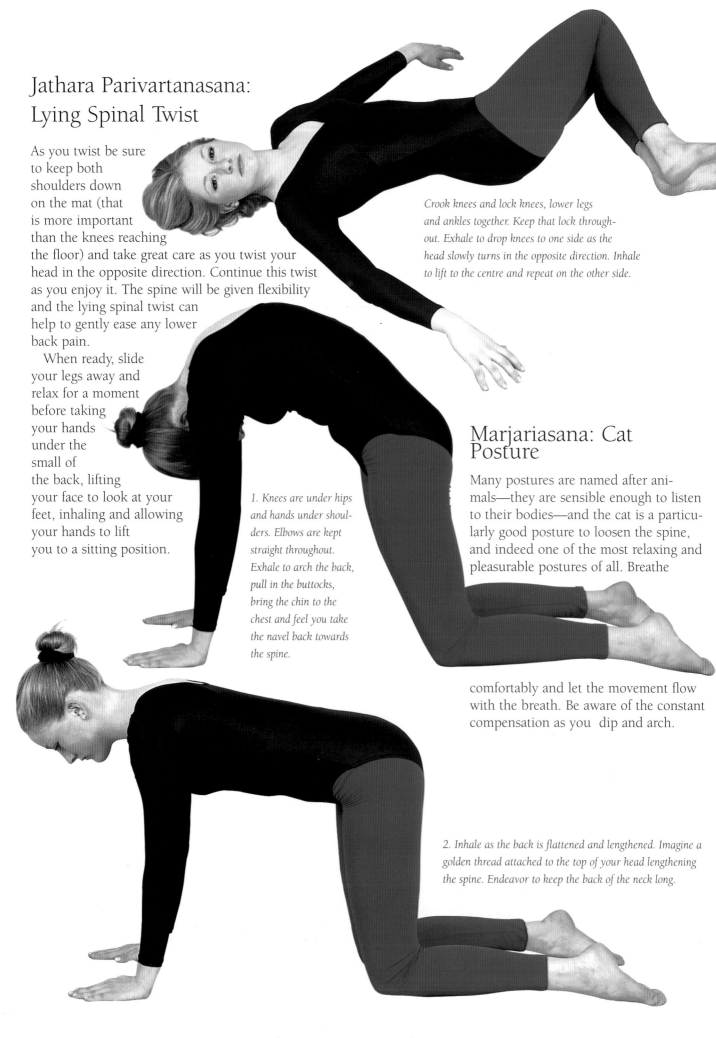

Jathara Parivartanasana: Lying Spinal Twist

As you twist be sure to keep both shoulders down on the mat (that is more important than the knees reaching the floor) and take great care as you twist your head in the opposite direction. Continue this twist as you enjoy it. The spine will be given flexibility and the lying spinal twist can help to gently ease any lower back pain.

When ready, slide your legs away and relax for a moment before taking your hands under the small of the back, lifting your face to look at your feet, inhaling and allowing your hands to lift you to a sitting position.

Crook knees and lock knees, lower legs and ankles together. Keep that lock throughout. Exhale to drop knees to one side as the head slowly turns in the opposite direction. Inhale to lift to the centre and repeat on the other side.

1. Knees are under hips and hands under shoulders. Elbows are kept straight throughout. Exhale to arch the back, pull in the buttocks, bring the chin to the chest and feel you take the navel back towards the spine.

Marjariasana: Cat Posture

Many postures are named after animals—they are sensible enough to listen to their bodies—and the cat is a particularly good posture to loosen the spine, and indeed one of the most relaxing and pleasurable postures of all. Breathe comfortably and let the movement flow with the breath. Be aware of the constant compensation as you dip and arch.

2. Inhale as the back is flattened and lengthened. Imagine a golden thread attached to the top of your head lengthening the spine. Endeavor to keep the back of the neck long.

14

Sphinx

Relax with your cheek on the mat and arms by your
sides and reflect on the constriction in the kidney
region experienced with the Sphinx.

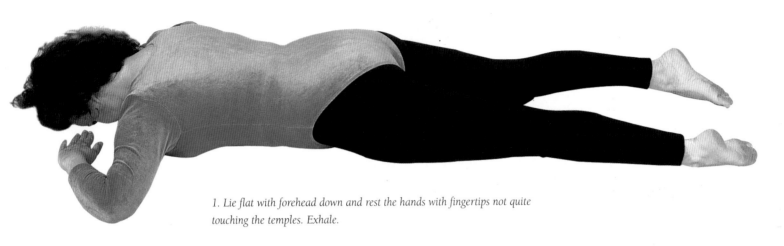

*1. Lie flat with forehead down and rest the hands with fingertips not quite
touching the temples. Exhale.*

*2. Inhale as head, shoulders and upper back lift off the mat to almost straighten
the elbows. Then simply swivel the palms until the elbows can rest underneath
the shoulders. Breathe normally in the posture, relaxing the shoulders and
keeping the neck long and in line with the spine. Inhale and lift elbows, swivel
palms and rest down where you began. Repeat twice.*

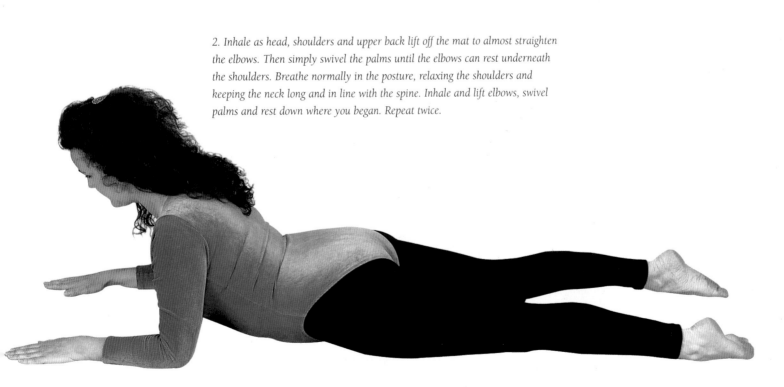

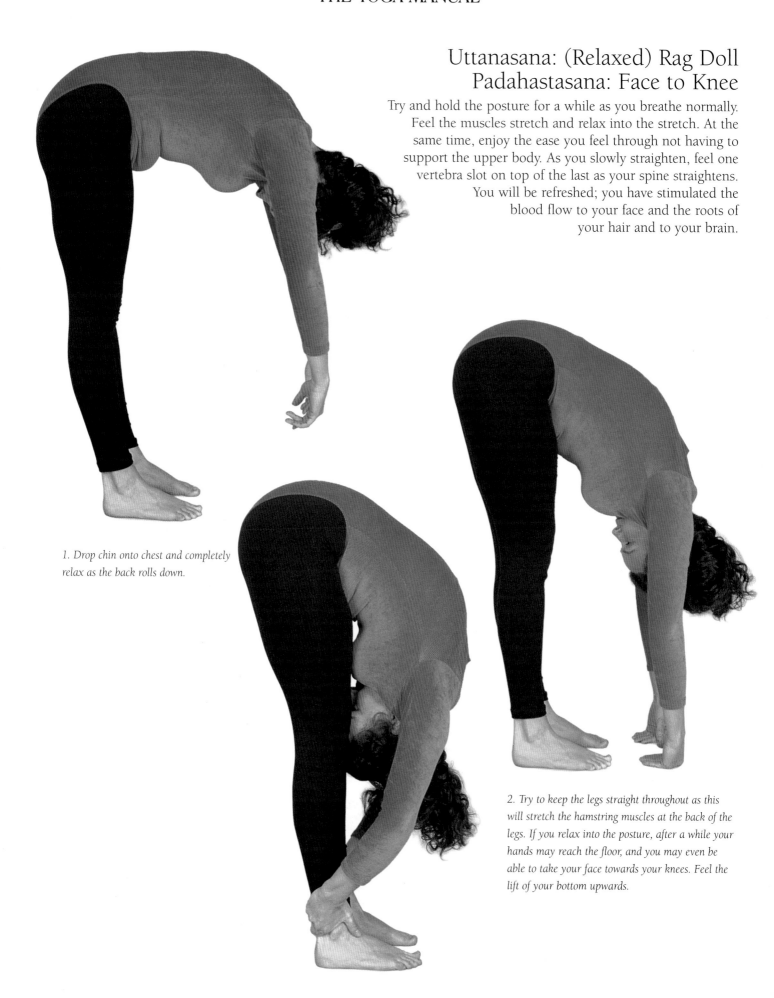

Uttanasana: (Relaxed) Rag Doll
Padahastasana: Face to Knee

Try and hold the posture for a while as you breathe normally. Feel the muscles stretch and relax into the stretch. At the same time, enjoy the ease you feel through not having to support the upper body. As you slowly straighten, feel one vertebra slot on top of the last as your spine straightens. You will be refreshed; you have stimulated the blood flow to your face and the roots of your hair and to your brain.

1. Drop chin onto chest and completely relax as the back rolls down.

2. Try to keep the legs straight throughout as this will stretch the hamstring muscles at the back of the legs. If you relax into the posture, after a while your hands may reach the floor, and you may even be able to take your face towards your knees. Feel the lift of your bottom upwards.

16

Standing Stretch

Don't look up at your hands as you work as this will compress the back of your neck.

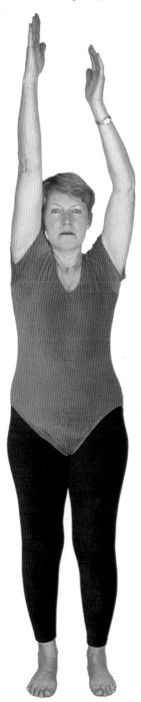

Twist

It is conventional to twist towards the end of a Yoga session as this centers the body and aligns the spine. Always be still for a moment after a twist to consolidate this centering.

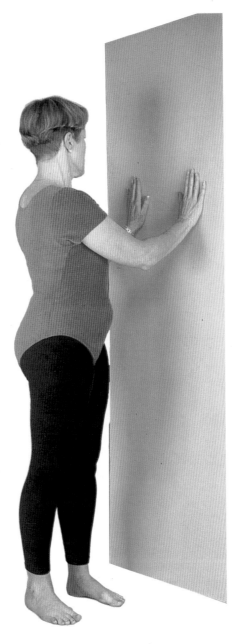

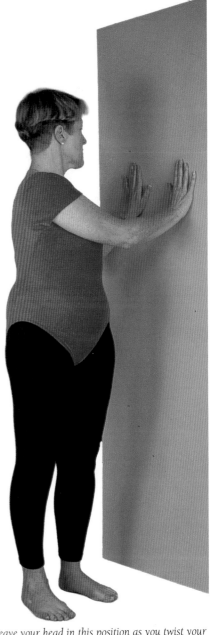

Ensure the feet are under the hips and parallel. Inhale to stretch through one side. Exhale, relaxing the stretch and repeat on the other side. Stretch three times on each side.

1. Stand about one foot (thirty centimeters) from the wall at a ninety-degree angle to it. Rest palms against the wall, with your face looking towards them.

2. Leave your head in this position as you twist your hips round towards the same direction as the feet. Feel the twist below the shoulder blades as you relax the shoulders and breathe normally in the posture. Slouch out of it when you are ready and turn to face the other direction to repeat.

Vrksasana: Tree Balance

We end the movement part of our Yoga with a balance posture which will aid the circulation and co-ordination and induce a feeling of harmony.

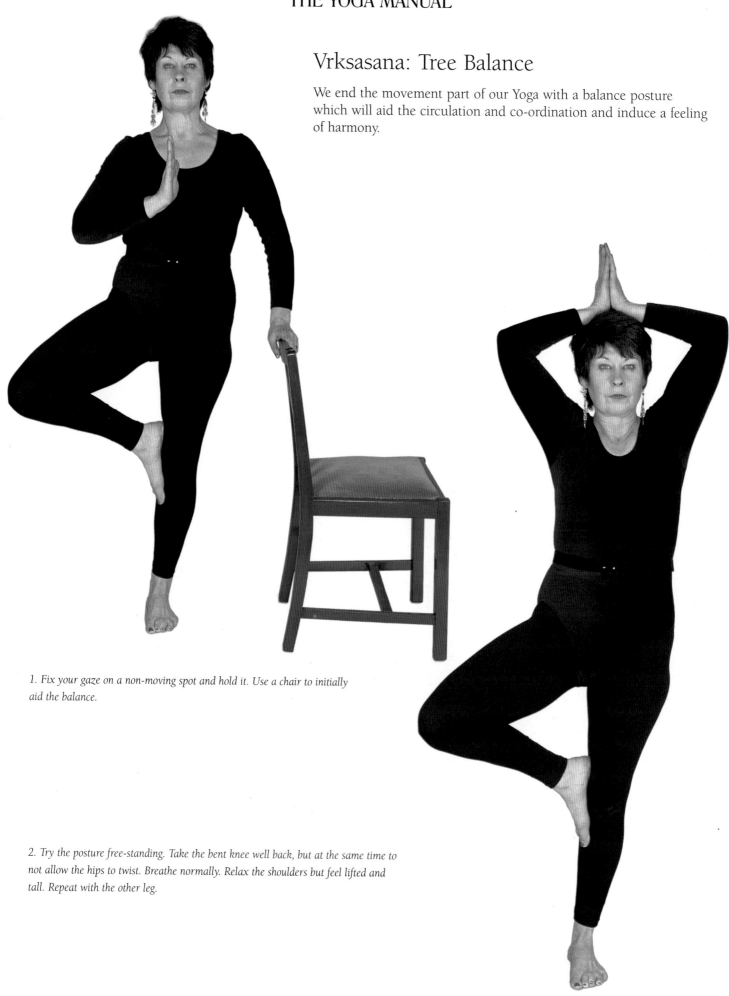

1. Fix your gaze on a non-moving spot and hold it. Use a chair to initially aid the balance.

2. Try the posture free-standing. Take the bent knee well back, but at the same time to not allow the hips to twist. Breathe normally. Relax the shoulders but feel lifted and tall. Repeat with the other leg.

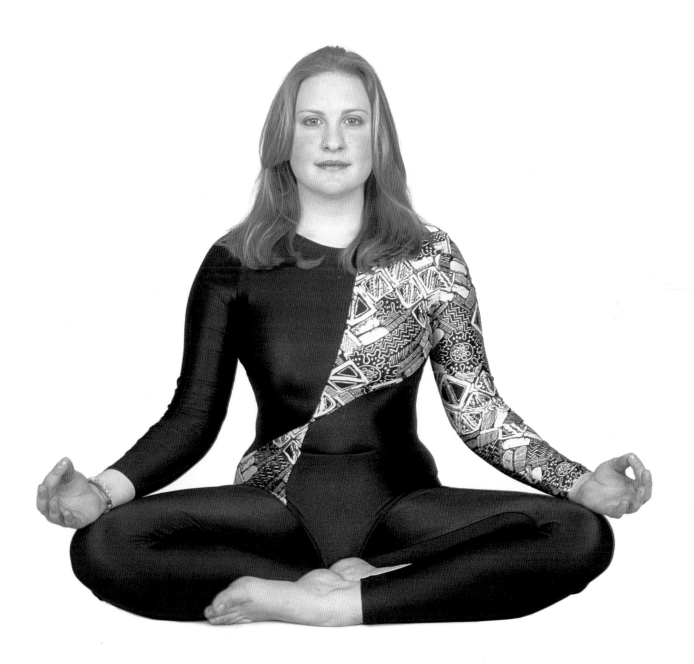

Pranayama: Yoga Breathing (Ratio Breath)

The breath retention, even for a short time, ensures that the prana or vital life-force breathed, is stored in the body for future use. Also, any breath which has a longer exhalation is calming.

It may be more comfortable to sit in a slightly raised position, for example on a book or a thin cushion placed under the sitting bones, or indeed with your back against a wall.

Sit either cross-legged or with heels in line with the perineum, hands resting palms uppermost and with thumb and forefinger meeting. The back is straight and the eyes closed. Allow the body and breath to become relaxed and comfortable. Begin Pranayama breathing in to a count of four, holding for a count of two, exhaling to a count of six. Breathe six breaths in this way.

Yoga Nidra: Total Relaxation

Enjoy lying down and relaxing as at the beginning of your Yoga. Always end your Yoga with this total relaxation—it will remove the fatigue caused by the postures and calm the mind. At the same time, the stretching and concentration of your Yoga have prepared the body and mind for relaxation.

Let go the shoulders, gently roll the neck from side to side. As your breath becomes calm and slow, your back will flatten into the mat. Tense the muscles in the legs and feet and see how relaxed they feel as you let go the tension. Do the same with the arms and hands. Allow the fingers to curl naturally. Your abdomen rises and falls almost imperceptibly with the breath. Your face is relaxed as you let go the tension at the bridge of your nose, your forehead and jaw. Your eyes will feel soft and seem to sink back into your head. You feel very heavy. Your body seems to sink into the floor. You are relaxed. Simply enjoy the peace and calm as you let the music softly float through your mind and your breath flow through your body.

When you are ready to come out of your relaxation, allow the breath to begin to deepen and bring your senses back into the room. Begin to move a little, perhaps just beginning with fingers and toes, working towards a long stretch and yawn. Roll over onto your right side for a while to take the strain off your heart before sitting up and opening your eyes.

When the five senses and the mind are still, and reason itself rests in silence, then begins the path supreme. This calm steadiness of the senses is called Yoga.

—From *The Katha Upanishad*

Opposite: Face to knee posture.

Below: Always end your Yoga with this total relaxation—it will remove the fatigue caused by the postures and calm the mind.

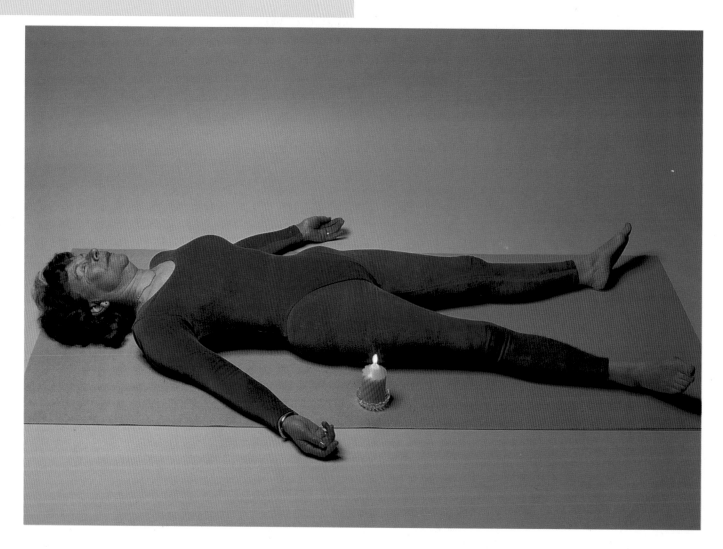

20

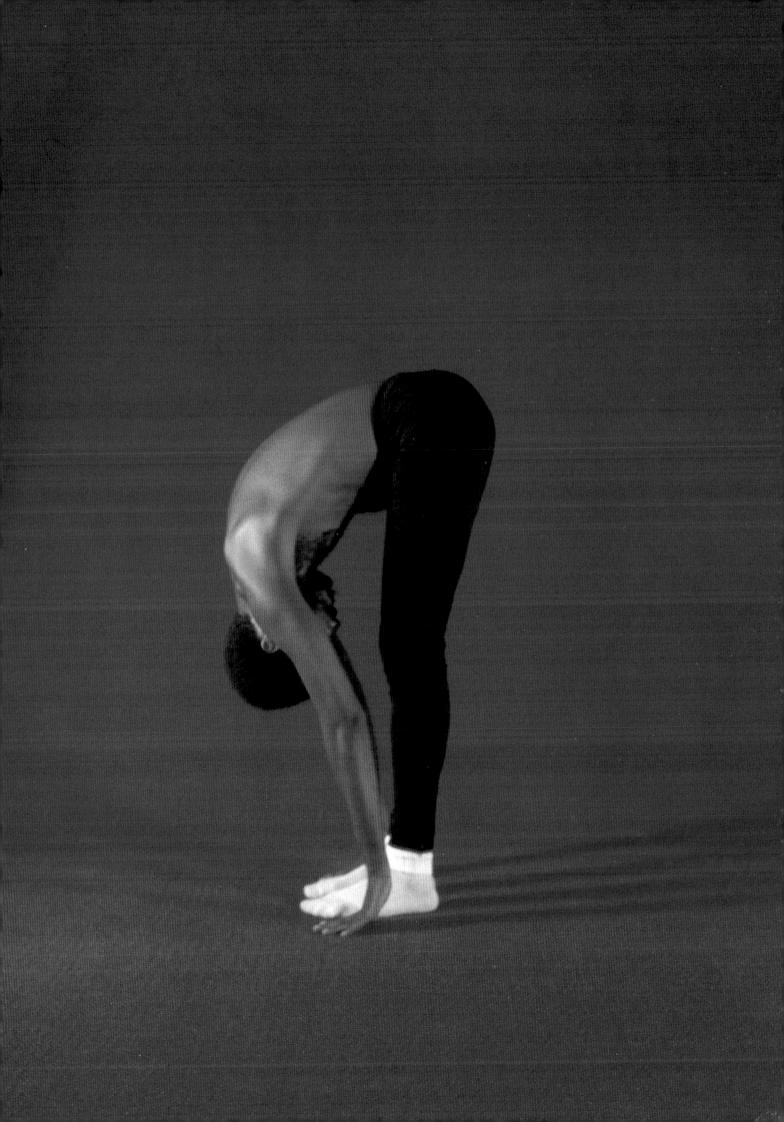

CHAPTER TWO

MORE STRETCH OF THE SPINE

This chapter will continue the stretch of the spine and begin to open the hip joints and pelvic region, which will also help the lengthening of the spine.

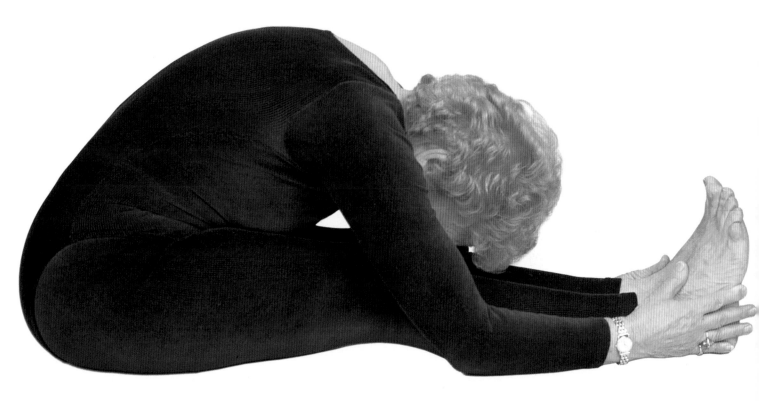

Savasana: Relaxation

Rest down and allow yourself to become calm and comfortable. Be aware of any sounds and sensations around you and as you become relaxed you will find you seem to become further and further removed from them, they are less and less important—the only really important thing now is for you to relax and sink down into the floor.

We choose our next world through what we learn in this one. Learn nothing, and the next world is the same as this one, all the same limitations and lead weights to overcome.
—From *Jonathan Livingston Seagull* by Richard Bach

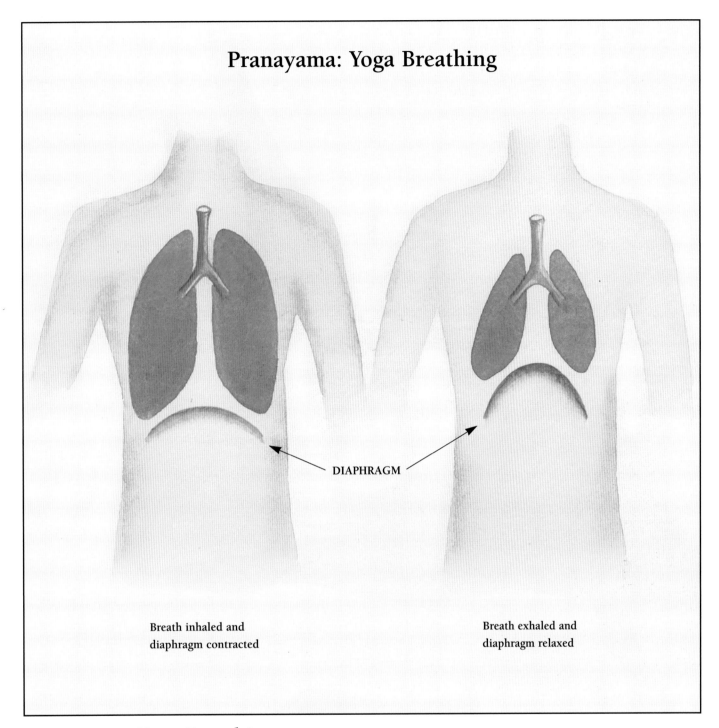

Pranayama: Yoga Breathing

DIAPHRAGM

Breath inhaled and
diaphragm contracted

Breath exhaled and
diaphragm relaxed

Pranayama: Yoga Breathing

Allow your consciousness to rest on your breath and
become aware of it as it flows through your body. Then
take that awareness to the diaphragm (the sheet of muscle below the lungs which separates the chest from the
abdomen) and watch as it contracts downwards with the
inhalation and so inflation of the lungs, and is allowed to
rise and relax as the lungs empty and so deflate. By doing
this you are allowing your thoughts to rest simply on
your breath. Relax that vision of the moving diaphragm
after a while and begin to move with a stretch and curl.

Leg Over Twisting Posture

If you wish, stay in the most dynamic part of the posture
and allow the weight of the leg to drop the foot a little
closer towards the floor. Continue to breathe comfortably.

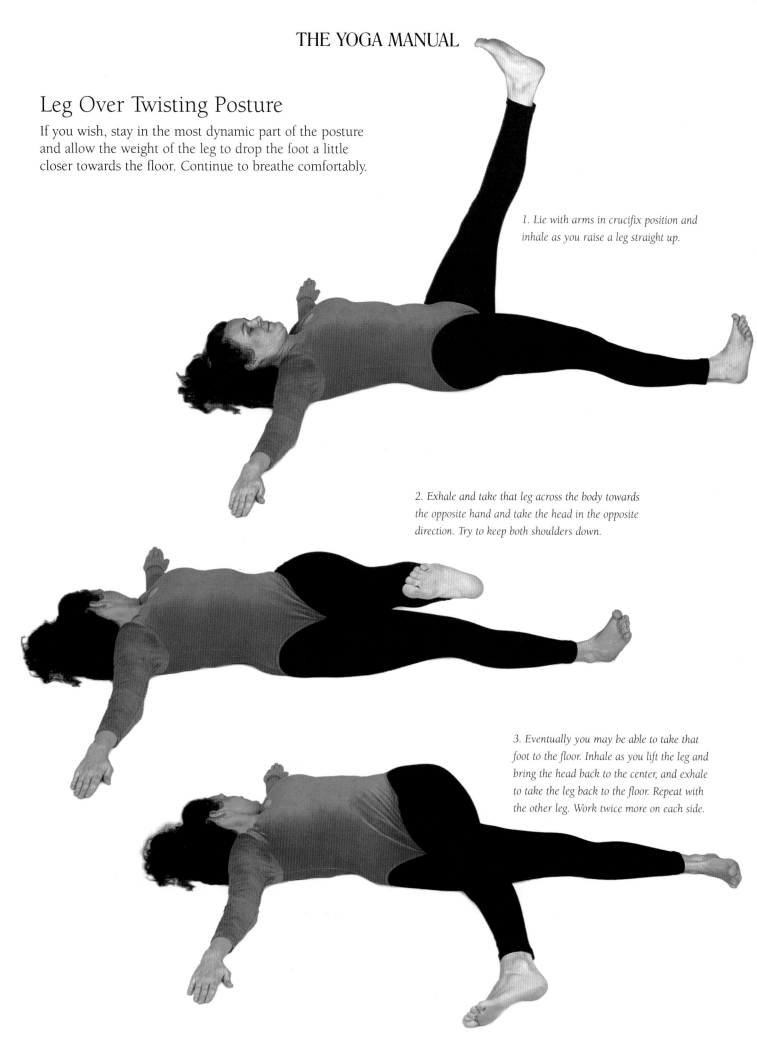

*1. Lie with arms in crucifix position and
inhale as you raise a leg straight up.*

*2. Exhale and take that leg across the body towards
the opposite hand and take the head in the opposite
direction. Try to keep both shoulders down.*

*3. Eventually you may be able to take that
foot to the floor. Inhale as you lift the leg and
bring the head back to the center, and exhale
to take the leg back to the floor. Repeat with
the other leg. Work twice more on each side.*

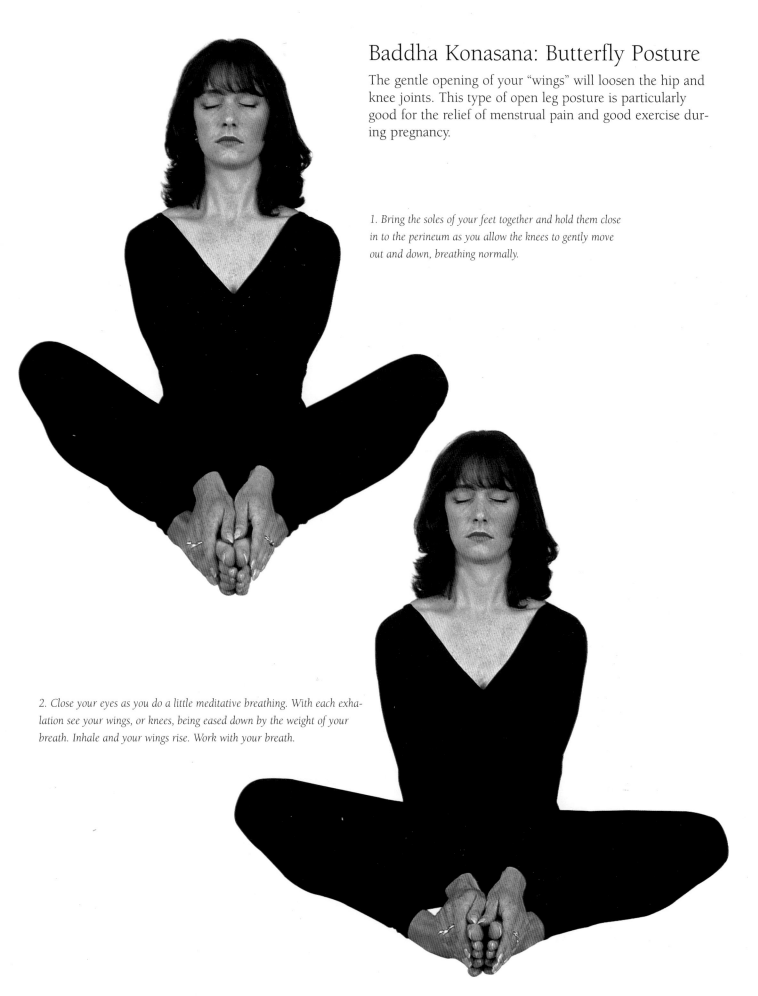

Baddha Konasana: Butterfly Posture

The gentle opening of your "wings" will loosen the hip and knee joints. This type of open leg posture is particularly good for the relief of menstrual pain and good exercise during pregnancy.

1. Bring the soles of your feet together and hold them close in to the perineum as you allow the knees to gently move out and down, breathing normally.

2. Close your eyes as you do a little meditative breathing. With each exhalation see your wings, or knees, being eased down by the weight of your breath. Inhale and your wings rise. Work with your breath.

Inward Roll of the Hips

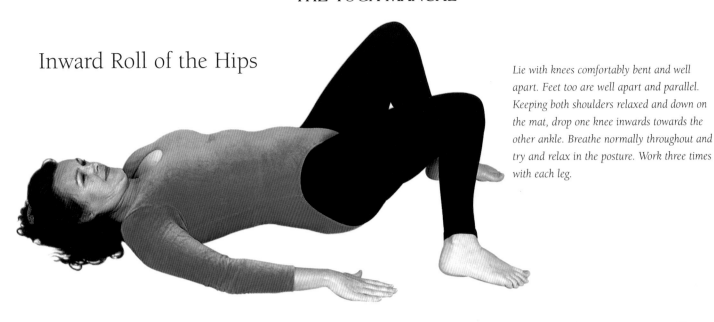

Lie with knees comfortably bent and well apart. Feet too are well apart and parallel. Keeping both shoulders relaxed and down on the mat, drop one knee inwards towards the other ankle. Breathe normally throughout and try and relax in the posture. Work three times with each leg.

Dog at Lampost

This posture will stretch the hip joint in the opposite dierction.

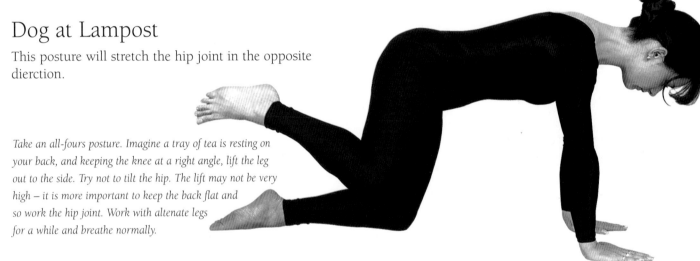

Take an all-fours posture. Imagine a tray of tea is resting on your back, and keeping the knee at a right angle, lift the leg out to the side. Try not to tilt the hip. The lift may not be very high – it is more important to keep the back flat and so work the hip joint. Work with altenate legs for a while and breathe normally.

Simhasana: Lion

In general we breath through the nose in Yoga, but there are a series of cleansing breaths such as The Lion, when we exhale throught the mouth.

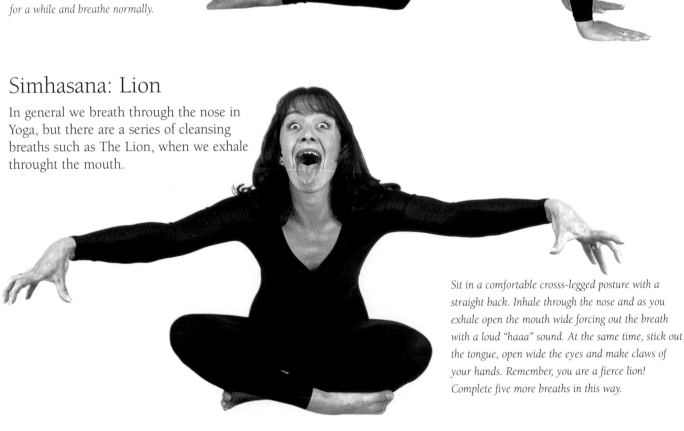

Sit in a comfortable crosss-legged posture with a straight back. Inhale through the nose and as you exhale open the mouth wide forcing out the breath with a loud "haaa" sound. At the same time, stick out the tongue, open wide the eyes and make claws of your hands. Remember, you are a fierce lion! Complete five more breaths in this way.

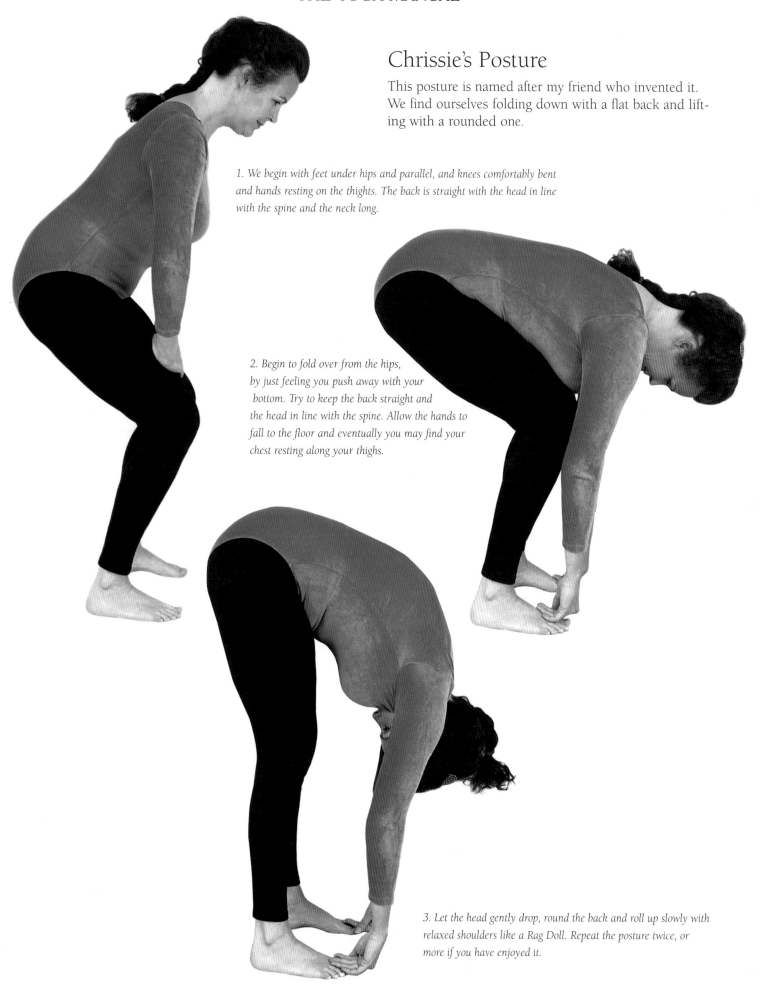

Chrissie's Posture

This posture is named after my friend who invented it. We find ourselves folding down with a flat back and lifting with a rounded one.

1. We begin with feet under hips and parallel, and knees comfortably bent and hands resting on the thights. The back is straight with the head in line with the spine and the neck long.

2. Begin to fold over from the hips, by just feeling you push away with your bottom. Try to keep the back straight and the head in line with the spine. Allow the hands to fall to the floor and eventually you may find your chest resting along your thighs.

3. Let the head gently drop, round the back and roll up slowly with relaxed shoulders like a Rag Doll. Repeat the posture twice, or more if you have enjoyed it.

Merudandasana: Coccyx Balance

The spot of balance may seem small, but persevere and it will come. The posture will help to improve your powers of concentration. Be sure there is room at your back to tuck your chin in and roll back if you loose your balance.

1. Sit well up on the sitting bones and draw the soles of the feet together. If possible, hook the forfingers round the big toes – if that is not possible, hold onto your ankles.

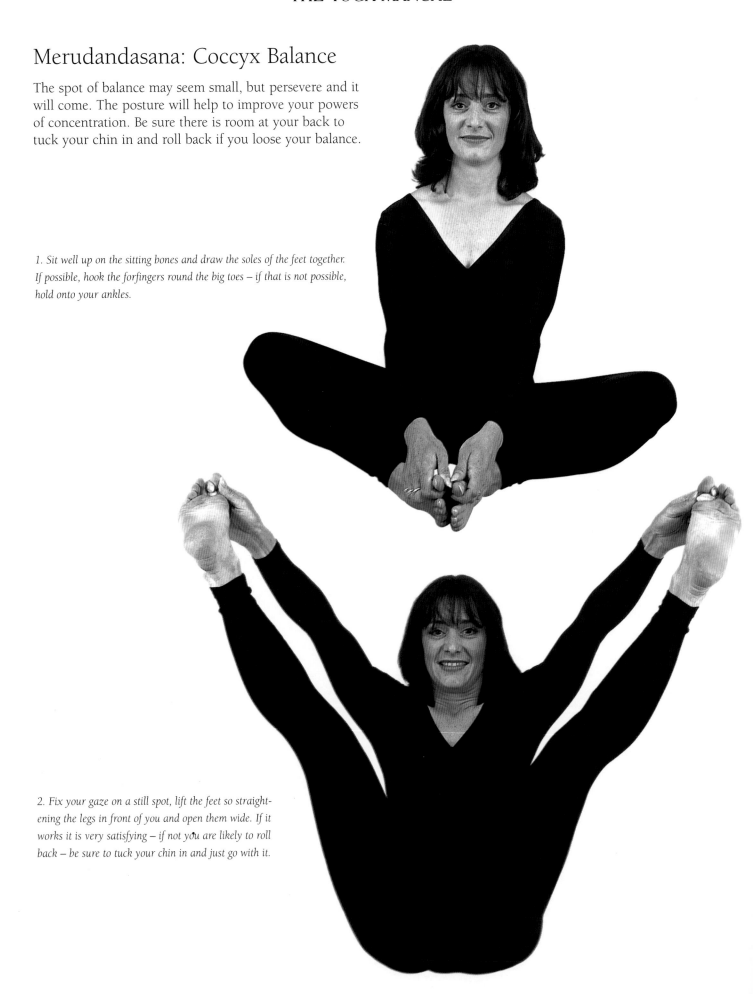

2. Fix your gaze on a still spot, lift the feet so straightening the legs in front of you and open them wide. If it works it is very satisfying – if not you are likely to roll back – be sure to tuck your chin in and just go with it.

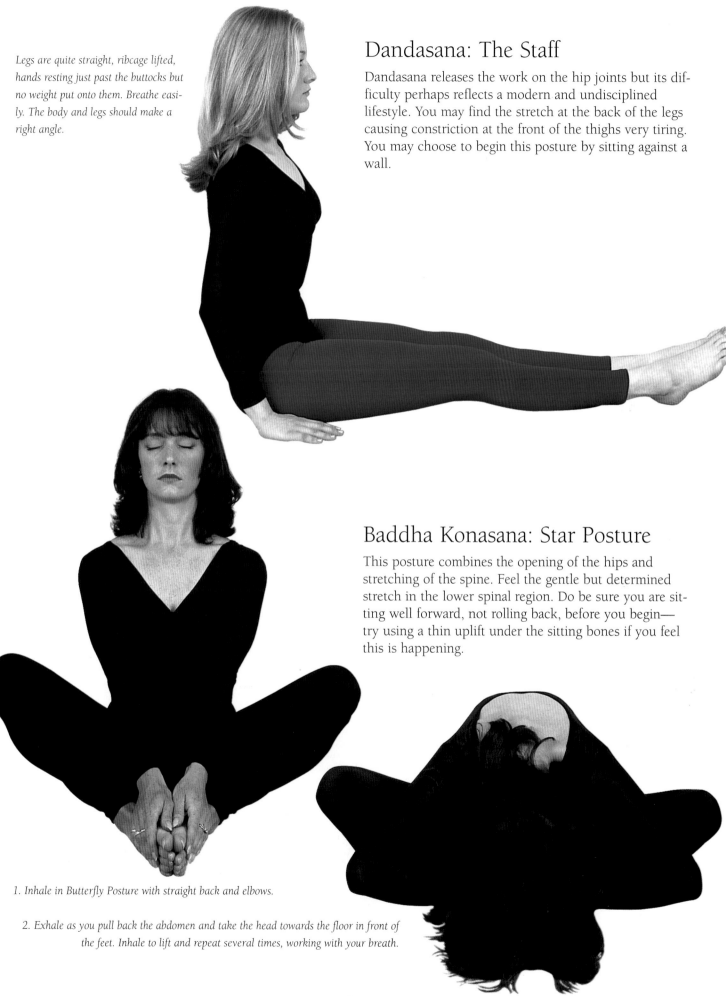

Legs are quite straight, ribcage lifted, hands resting just past the buttocks but no weight put onto them. Breathe easily. The body and legs should make a right angle.

Dandasana: The Staff

Dandasana releases the work on the hip joints but its difficulty perhaps reflects a modern and undisciplined lifestyle. You may find the stretch at the back of the legs causing constriction at the front of the thighs very tiring. You may choose to begin this posture by sitting against a wall.

Baddha Konasana: Star Posture

This posture combines the opening of the hips and stretching of the spine. Feel the gentle but determined stretch in the lower spinal region. Do be sure you are sitting well forward, not rolling back, before you begin—try using a thin uplift under the sitting bones if you feel this is happening.

1. Inhale in Butterfly Posture with straight back and elbows.

2. Exhale as you pull back the abdomen and take the head towards the floor in front of the feet. Inhale to lift and repeat several times, working with your breath.

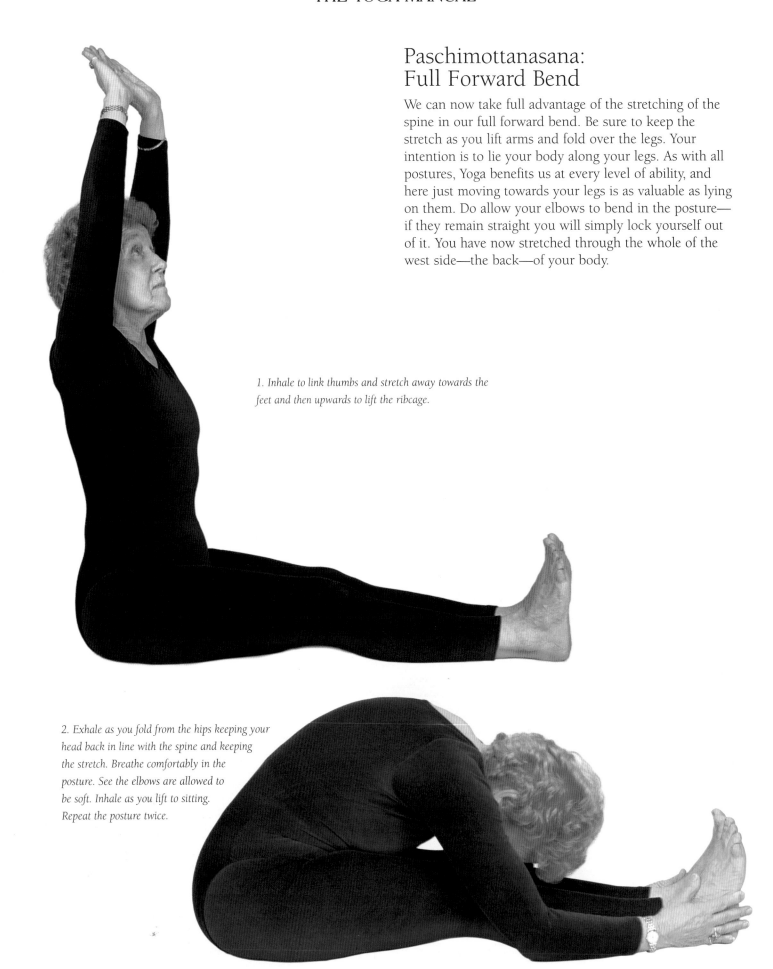

Paschimottanasana: Full Forward Bend

We can now take full advantage of the stretching of the spine in our full forward bend. Be sure to keep the stretch as you lift arms and fold over the legs. Your intention is to lie your body along your legs. As with all postures, Yoga benefits us at every level of ability, and here just moving towards your legs is as valuable as lying on them. Do allow your elbows to bend in the posture— if they remain straight you will simply lock yourself out of it. You have now stretched through the whole of the west side—the back—of your body.

1. Inhale to link thumbs and stretch away towards the feet and then upwards to lift the ribcage.

2. Exhale as you fold from the hips keeping your head back in line with the spine and keeping the stretch. Breathe comfortably in the posture. See the elbows are allowed to be soft. Inhale as you lift to sitting. Repeat the posture twice.

Backward Bend

Compensate with a backward bend.

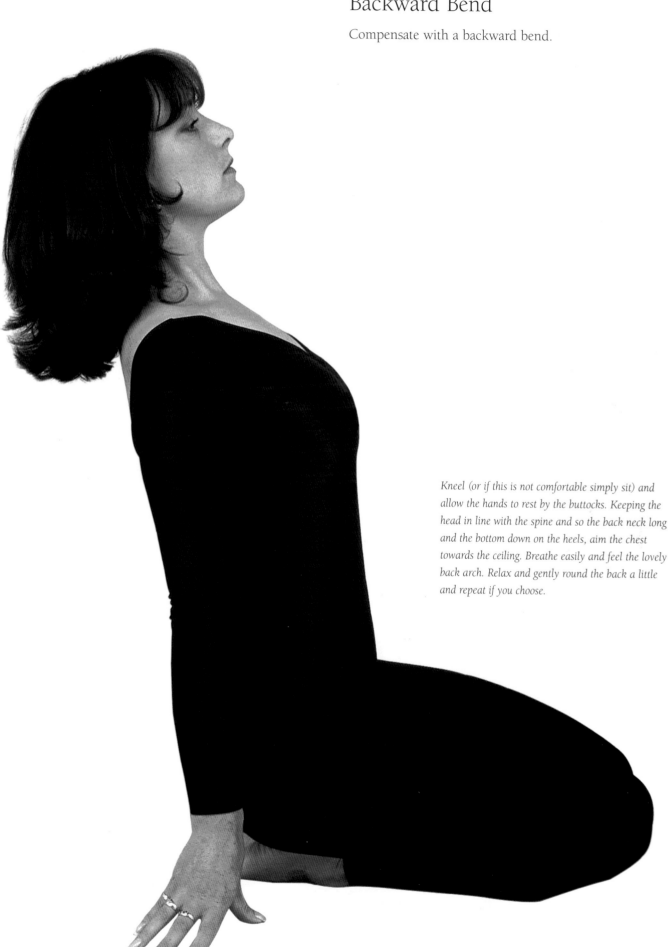

Kneel (or if this is not comfortable simply sit) and allow the hands to rest by the buttocks. Keeping the head in line with the spine and so the back neck long and the bottom down on the heels, aim the chest towards the ceiling. Breathe easily and feel the lovely back arch. Relax and gently round the back a little and repeat if you choose.

Bharadvajanasana: Twist in a Chair

1. Sit sideways on a chair and grasp the back of it with both hands. Take a breath in and lift the ribcage.

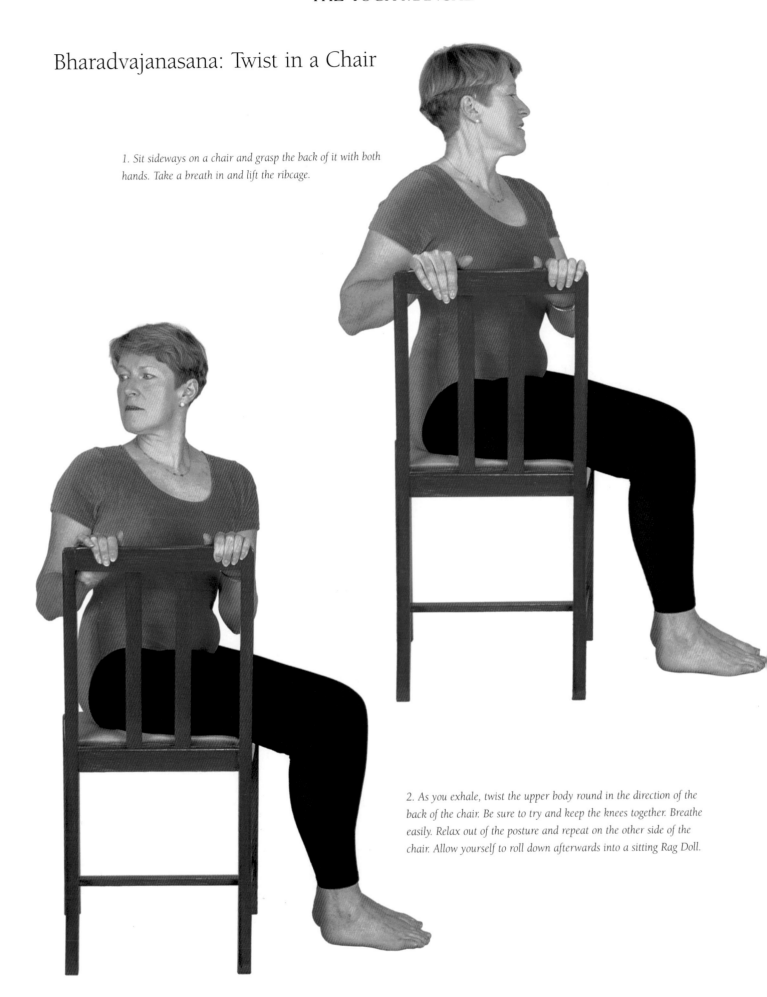

2. As you exhale, twist the upper body round in the direction of the back of the chair. Be sure to try and keep the knees together. Breathe easily. Relax out of the posture and repeat on the other side of the chair. Allow yourself to roll down afterwards into a sitting Rag Doll.

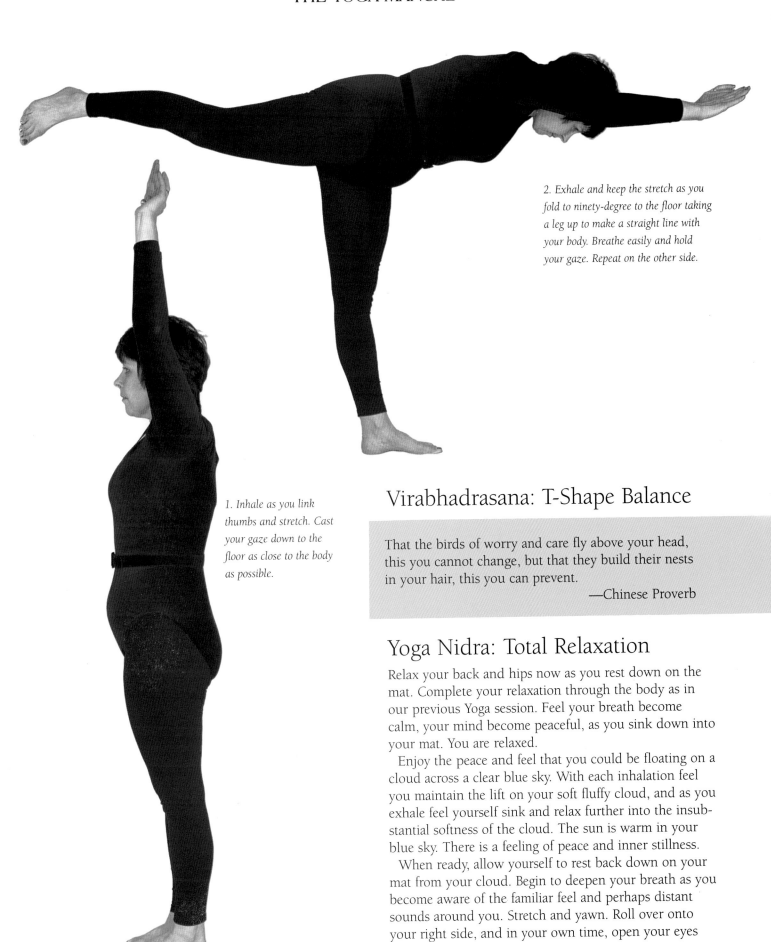

2. Exhale and keep the stretch as you fold to ninety-degree to the floor taking a leg up to make a straight line with your body. Breathe easily and hold your gaze. Repeat on the other side.

1. Inhale as you link thumbs and stretch. Cast your gaze down to the floor as close to the body as possible.

Virabhadrasana: T-Shape Balance

That the birds of worry and care fly above your head, this you cannot change, but that they build their nests in your hair, this you can prevent.

—Chinese Proverb

Yoga Nidra: Total Relaxation

Relax your back and hips now as you rest down on the mat. Complete your relaxation through the body as in our previous Yoga session. Feel your breath become calm, your mind become peaceful, as you sink down into your mat. You are relaxed.

Enjoy the peace and feel that you could be floating on a cloud across a clear blue sky. With each inhalation feel you maintain the lift on your soft fluffy cloud, and as you exhale feel yourself sink and relax further into the insubstantial softness of the cloud. The sun is warm in your blue sky. There is a feeling of peace and inner stillness.

When ready, allow yourself to rest back down on your mat from your cloud. Begin to deepen your breath as you become aware of the familiar feel and perhaps distant sounds around you. Stretch and yawn. Roll over onto your right side, and in your own time, open your eyes and sit up.

CHAPTER THREE

OPENING
THE HIPS

*This Yoga session will build on the opening of the hip joints,
flatten the back, and increase the strength of the legs.*

Just for today I will have
a program. I may not fol-
low it exactly, but I will
have it. I will save myself
from two pests: hurry
and indecision.

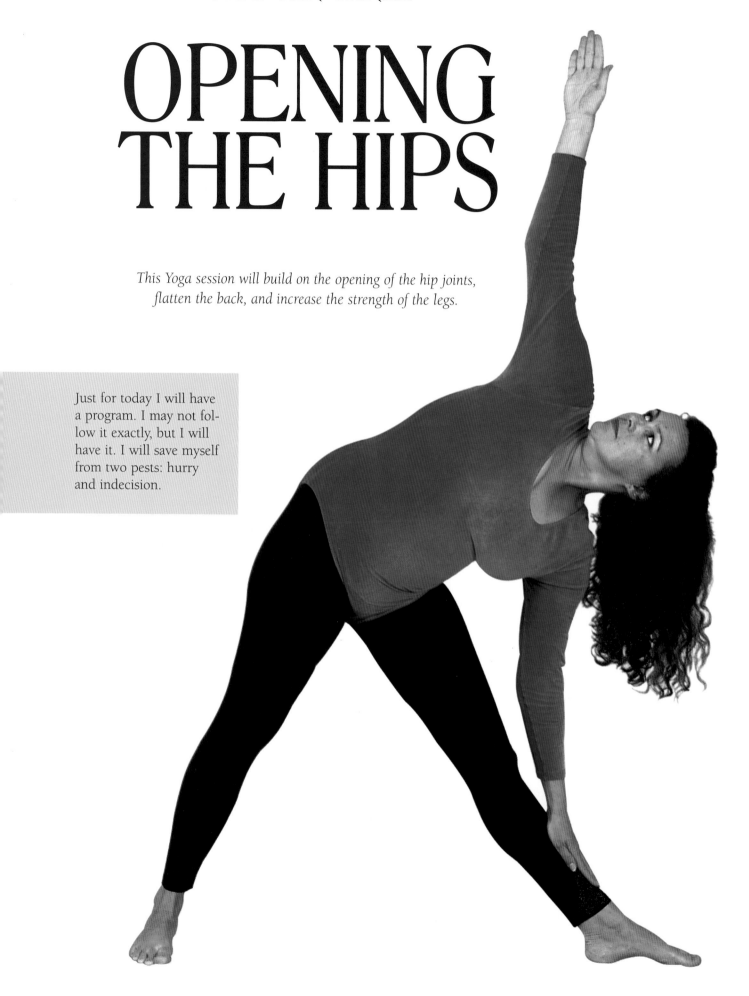

Begin in Savasana for a quiet start to your Yoga. Relax into the mat and allow the breath to become calm. Release the tension and as you breath, with each exhalation repeat to yourself the mantra (or repetition) "let go."

Pranayama Yoga Breathing

Abdominal Breathing: Inhale through the nose and fill the lower part of the lungs—feel the abdominal wall arch outwards. The lower part of the lungs only fill and the chest and shoulders remain motionless. As you exhale, feel the abdominal wall drawn in. Repeat four times.

Middle Breathing: Direct the breath to the middle part of the chest. Inhale and expand the ribs to both sides. The abdomen and shoulders remain motionless as only the mid-lungs fill with air. Exhale and feel the ribs contract. Repeat four times.

Upper Breathing: Inhale into the top of the lungs, lifting the collar-bone and shoulders. The abdomen and chest remain motionless. Exhale and lower the upper chest and shoulders. Repeat four times.

Relax and allow the breath to become normal before stretching and curling.

What we are today comes from our thoughts of yesterday, and our present thoughts build our life of tomorrow: our life is the creation of our mind.

If a man speaks or acts with an impure mind, suffering follows him as the wheel of the cart follows the beast that draws the cart.

If a man speaks or acts with a pure mind, joy follows him as his own shadow.
—*The Dhammapada*

Side Leg Raise

Ensure the hips are not twisted as you raise the leg. Let the lower leg be softly bent if that is more comfortable.

Arrange the body in a straight line, the elbow in line with the heels. Rest the other hand in front of the chest to balance. Exhale. Inhale and raise the top leg. Do not twist the hips. Exhale as the leg is lowered. Repeat twice, then roll onto the other side to work three times. Roll onto your back and relax for a while reflecting on the way the hips feel—one leg may have lifted higher than the other. You may well discover that the two sides of the body stretch differently in many postures.

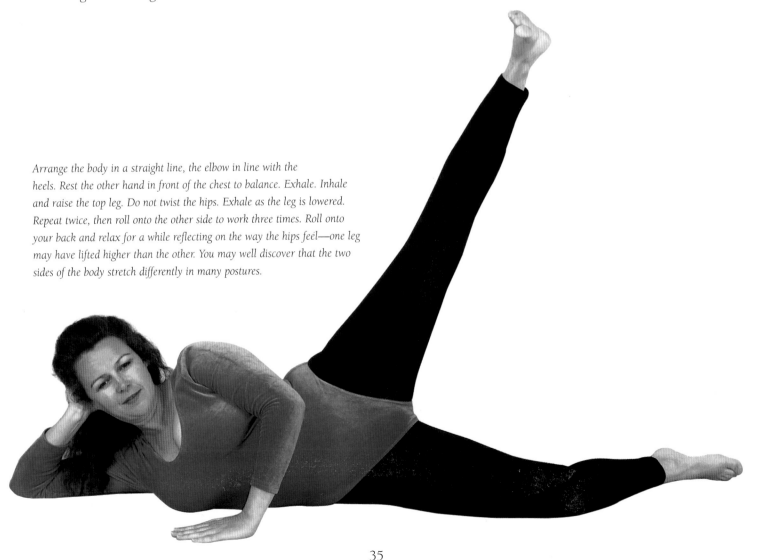

Ardha Padmasana: Half Lotus

If, when in the Half Lotus, the knee remains stubbornly high off the mat, place your hands on top of it and gently but firmly ease it down.

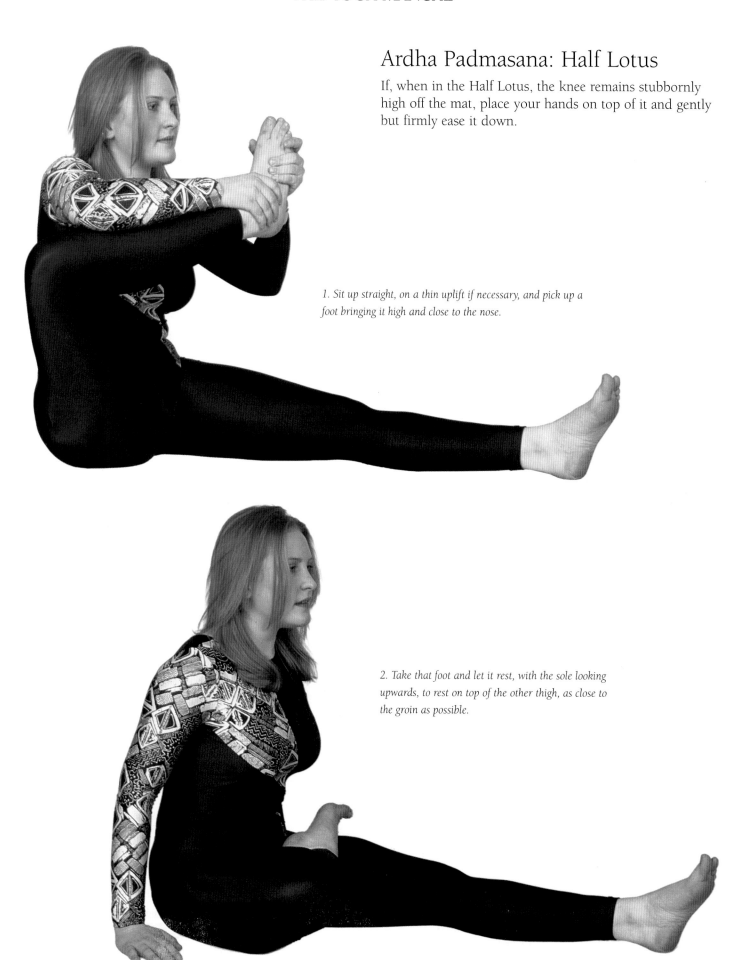

1. Sit up straight, on a thin uplift if necessary, and pick up a foot bringing it high and close to the nose.

2. Take that foot and let it rest, with the sole looking upwards, to rest on top of the other thigh, as close to the groin as possible.

Siamese Side Stretch

In the side stretch be sure to remain in a straight position with the head erect. You will not feel the stretch down the side of the body if you allow the head and shoulders to fall forward.

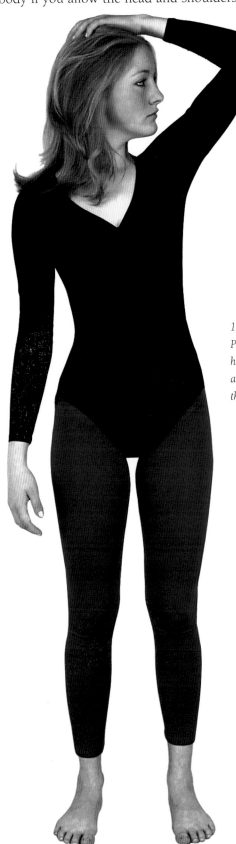

1. Stand with feet under hips. Place one hand on top of the head, take the elbow well back, and turn the head to look into the crook of that elbow. Inhale.

2. As you exhale, allow the other hand to slide down the thigh, thus taking the bent elbow upwards. Keep your gaze in the crook of the elbow. One side of the body will be stretched and the other constricted. Inhale as you slide that hand back up the thigh, and so bring the body back to a level position. Repeat twice. Then work three times on the other side.

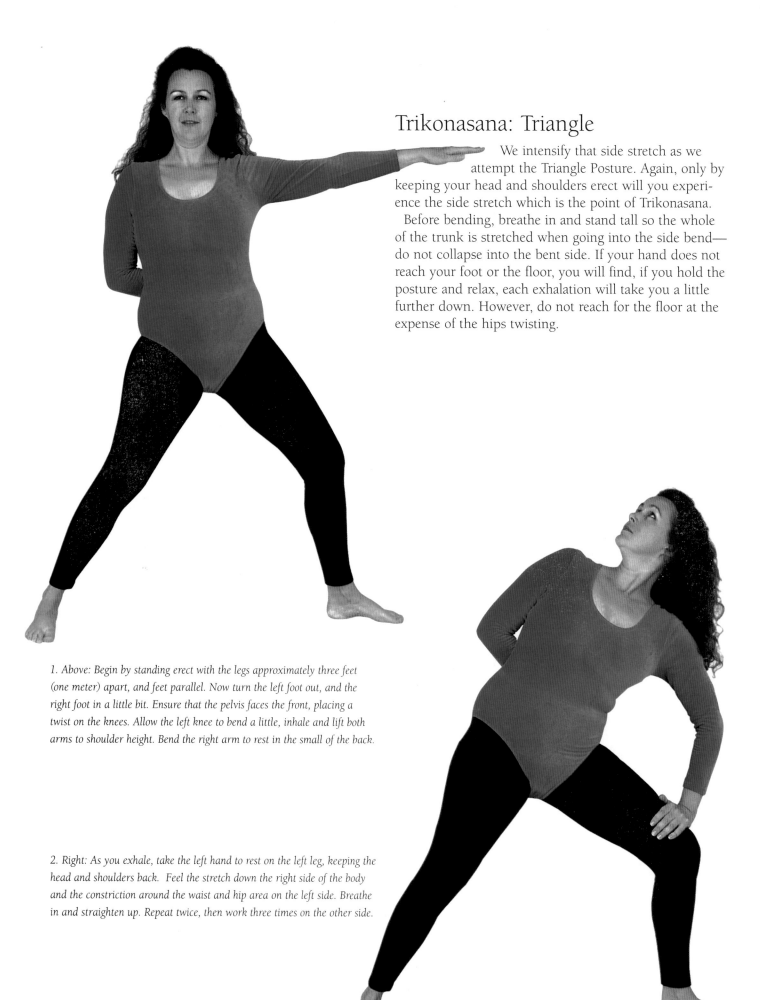

Trikonasana: Triangle

We intensify that side stretch as we attempt the Triangle Posture. Again, only by keeping your head and shoulders erect will you experience the side stretch which is the point of Trikonasana.

Before bending, breathe in and stand tall so the whole of the trunk is stretched when going into the side bend—do not collapse into the bent side. If your hand does not reach your foot or the floor, you will find, if you hold the posture and relax, each exhalation will take you a little further down. However, do not reach for the floor at the expense of the hips twisting.

1. Above: Begin by standing erect with the legs approximately three feet (one meter) apart, and feet parallel. Now turn the left foot out, and the right foot in a little bit. Ensure that the pelvis faces the front, placing a twist on the knees. Allow the left knee to bend a little, inhale and lift both arms to shoulder height. Bend the right arm to rest in the small of the back.

2. Right: As you exhale, take the left hand to rest on the left leg, keeping the head and shoulders back. Feel the stretch down the right side of the body and the constriction around the waist and hip area on the left side. Breathe in and straighten up. Repeat twice, then work three times on the other side.

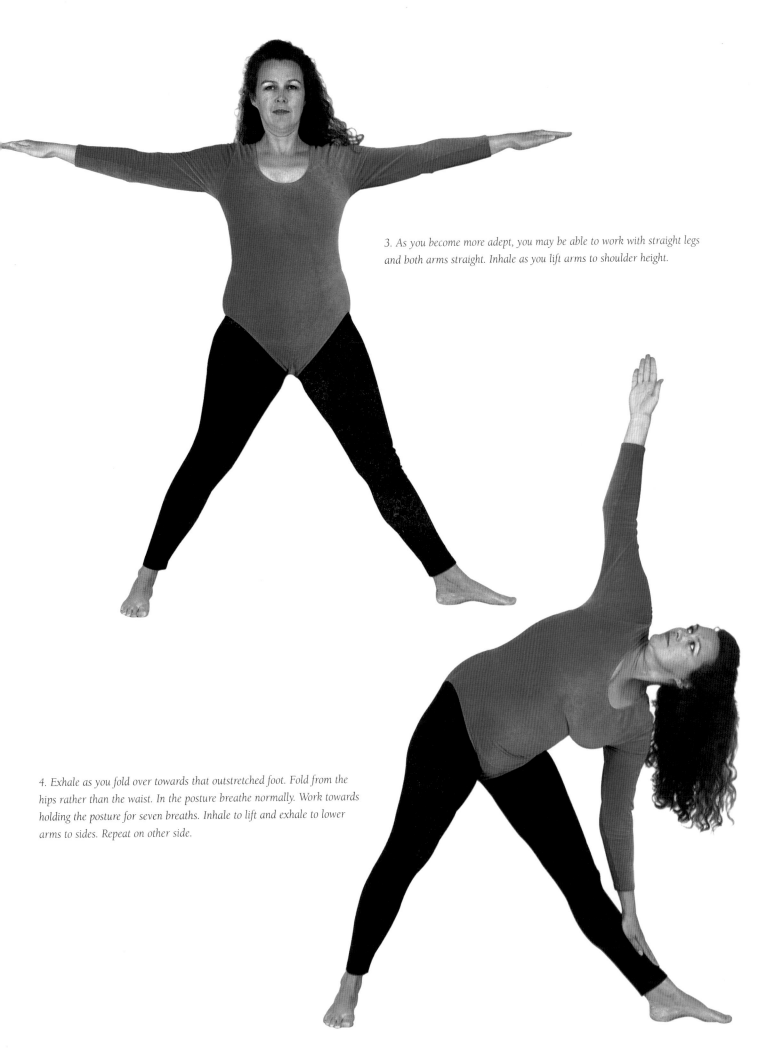

3. As you become more adept, you may be able to work with straight legs and both arms straight. Inhale as you lift arms to shoulder height.

4. Exhale as you fold over towards that outstretched foot. Fold from the hips rather than the waist. In the posture breathe normally. Work towards holding the posture for seven breaths. Inhale to lift and exhale to lower arms to sides. Repeat on other side.

Chest Expansion

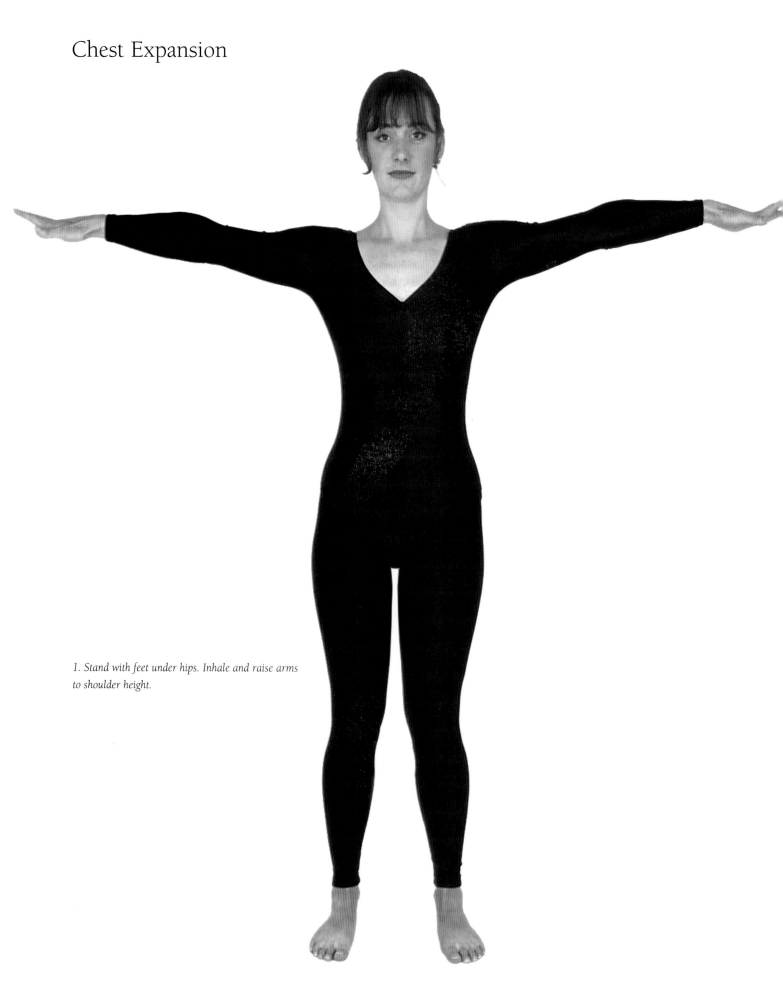

1. Stand with feet under hips. Inhale and raise arms to shoulder height.

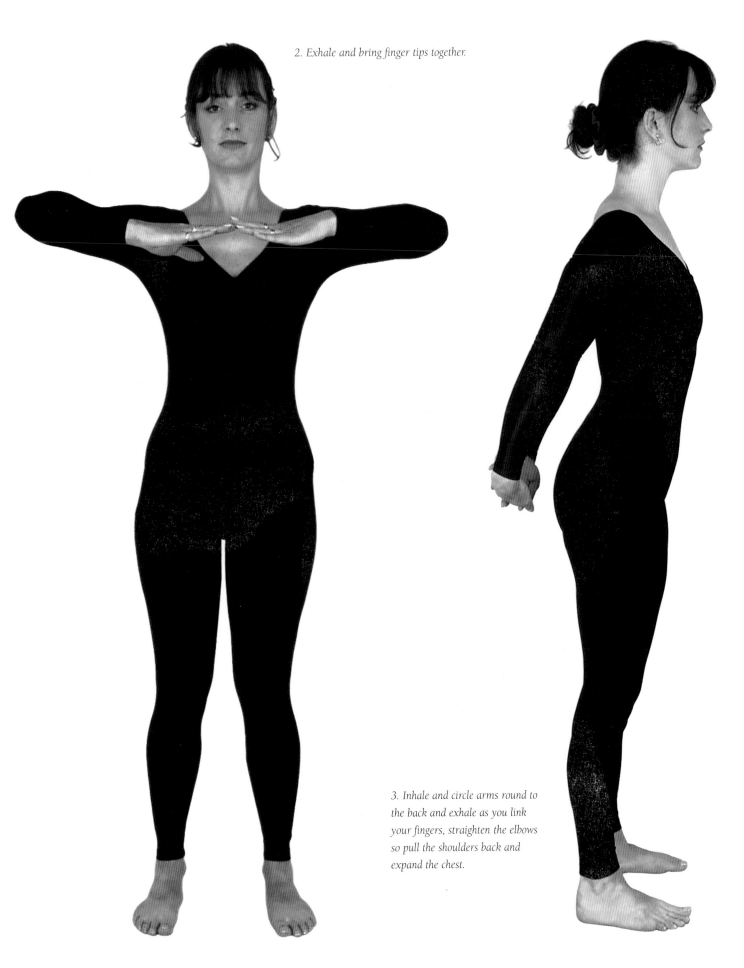

2. Exhale and bring finger tips together.

3. Inhale and circle arms round to the back and exhale as you link your fingers, straighten the elbows so pull the shoulders back and expand the chest.

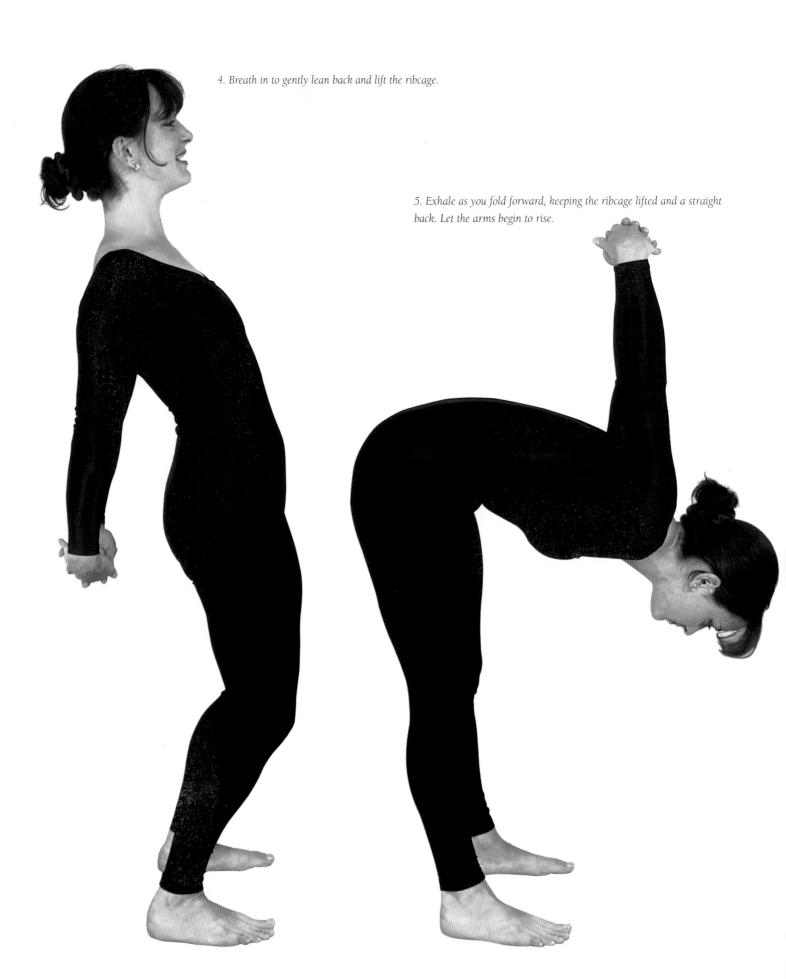

4. Breath in to gently lean back and lift the ribcage.

5. Exhale as you fold forward, keeping the ribcage lifted and a straight back. Let the arms begin to rise.

Floppy Twist

Plant the feet under the hips, take arms out to the front at shoulder height and just swing into a floppy twist. Let the whole of the body, including the head gently twist with the momentum, and don't suddenly stop, let it wind down – drop the car into neutral!

6. When you will not fold any further, let the head drop towards the knees, relaxing the shoulders so that the arms lift and maybe travel overhead towards the floor. Breathe normally in the posture. When ready to lift, raise the head first to straighten the spine, inhale and lift, until you are gently leaning back, as when going down into the posture. Exhale as you stand straight and release your hands. Repeat twice.

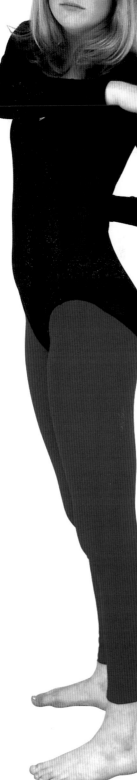

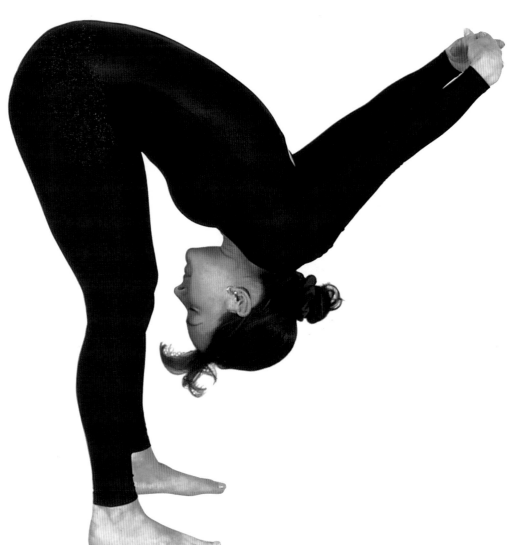

Uttanasana:
(Supported) Flat Back Stretch

If there are any lower back problems it is not good to work with both straight legs and straight back at the same time. If this is the case, let the knees be softly bent as you work. This advice applies to all flat back/straight leg postures.

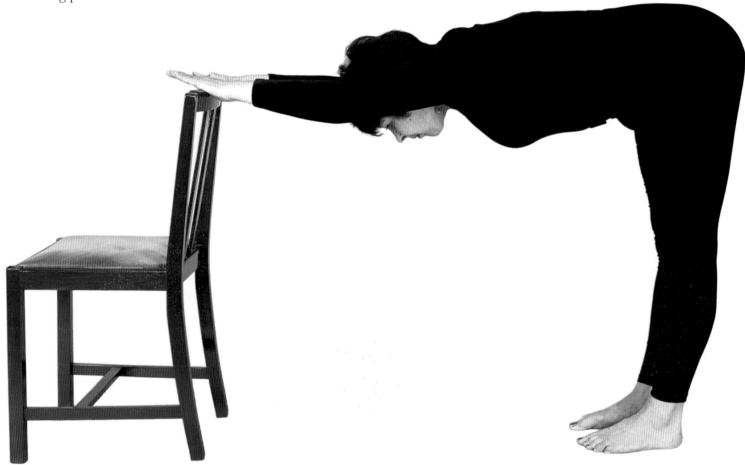

Inhale, linking thumbs and stretching tall. As you exhale push back on the knees and buttocks and fold forward, continuing to stretch. Allow the hands to rest, not letting the wrists droop, and keeping the ears close to inner arms. Try to flatten the back. Breathe easily. Either stretch out of the posture as you stretched in, or bend the knees and roll the back up to standing.

"Don't go outside your house to see the flowers.

My friend, don't bother with that excursion.

Inside your body there are flowers.

One has a thousand petals.

That will do for a place to sit.

Sitting there you will have a glimpse of beauty

inside the body and out of it,

before gardens and after gardens."

Kabir

Pranayama: Cooling Breath

This is a breath which will cool and refresh. Sit in a comfortable easy pose as in Pranayama at the end of Chapter One. Inhale through a tiny hole in almost closed lips, with the teeth just apart and the tip of the tongue close to the front teeth. Exhale through the nose. Work comfortably in this way with your breath, feeling the body become cool and the mind refreshed.

Yoga Nidra: Total Relaxation

To complete your Yoga lie down and slowly relax through the body. By now you will know which parts of your body tend to told onto tension—perhaps your forehead or shoulders. Allow no part of the body to be neglected. Notice how your body and mind take on a feeling of calm as you relax.

Visualize a warm red glow at the base of the spine. Feel the warmth and comfort from that glow seem to ease the base of the spine into the floor. Allow that red glow to spread through the rest of the body. As it spreads, the color becomes less intense, so that by the time it reaches the extremities it is quite pink. If, however, there are any parts of the body which need particular loving care and attention, deepen the color there and feel that with each exhalation you breath the warmth from your red glow into them to give warmth and comfort.

After a period of experiencing that warm glow through out, begin to allow it to shrink back to the lower spine and eventually to disappear altogether. You will feel warm, comforted and healed.

When you are ready, begin to deepen the breath, and stretch and yawn before rolling over onto the right side and coming up to sitting.

CHAPTER FOUR
INVERTED POSTURES

In this session we shall be putting some thought to inverted postures. These postures will improve the circulation, especially in the legs and stomach, and improve the flow of blood to the brain through action on the thyroid gland.

Just for today I will be unafraid. Especially I will not be afraid to enjoy what is beautiful, and to believe that as I give to the world, so the world will give to me.

Begin in Savasana. Relax down and give your body and mind that precious time to be calm. Sink into your mat and let go tension. Let your mind rest on a sound you may be able to hear—perhaps a bird outside, the murmur of voices in another room, the ticking of a clock—your thoughts seem to float around that sound.

After a few minutes, bring your awareness back to your body and breath. Gently let your breath deepen in preparation for Pranayama.

Pranayama Complete Yoga Breath

Feel the breath comfortable and easy. Visualize the navel and bring the concentration approximately 2 inches (5cm) above it. Begin to inhale, feeling you fill the lungs from this point up. As the lower then upper chest inflates, the ribcage will widen, the chest lift and the shoulders lift. You should endeavor to keep the abdomen flat throughout.

Exhale emptying the chest from the top down – the upper chest empties, the ribs contract and the lower chest relaxes. Repeat twice, making each breath as deep and long as feels right for you.

Be aware of that moment of involuntary hesitation before each exhalation and inhalation.

Relax and allow your breath to return to normal before you stretch and curl.

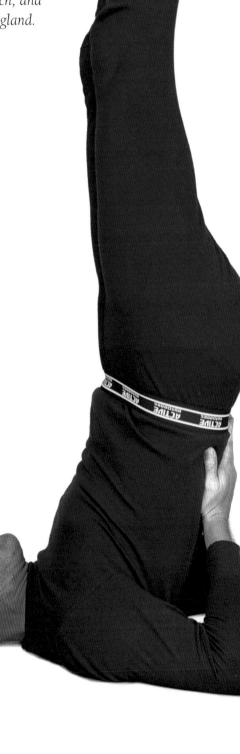

Padangusthasana: Toe Catch

If you can reach your feet try to link the index fingers around the big toes—this can help to ease straightness into that joint and correct any damage caused by ill-fitting shoes.

When you work as you are a flute through whose heart the whispering of the hours turns to music. Which of you would be a reed, dumb and silent, when all else sings together in unison?
—From *The Prophet* by Kahlil Gibran

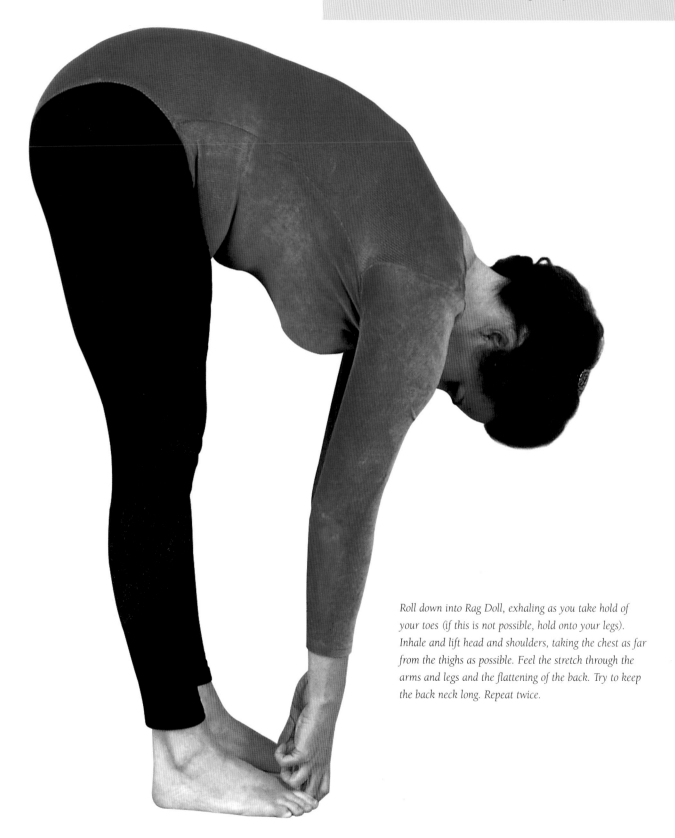

Roll down into Rag Doll, exhaling as you take hold of your toes (if this is not possible, hold onto your legs). Inhale and lift head and shoulders, taking the chest as far from the thighs as possible. Feel the stretch through the arms and legs and the flattening of the back. Try to keep the back neck long. Repeat twice.

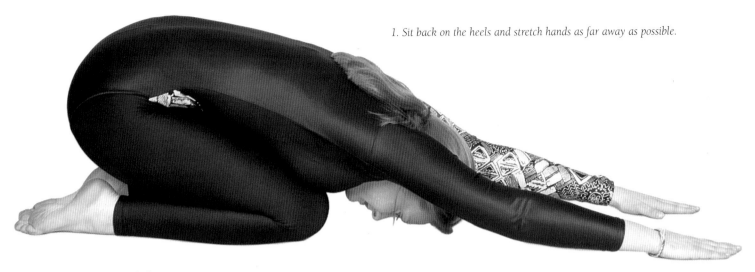

1. Sit back on the heels and stretch hands as far away as possible.

Adho Mukha Svanasana: Dog Posture

The stretch on the back of the legs in the toe catch prepares them for the same sensation in the Dog.

Feel the exhilaration of the stretch in the Dog. Use the whole of your hands, with fingers wide spread to push against. Imagine a hand gently pushing on the spine between the shoulder blades easing the chest back to the knees. Keep the arms straight throughout, but you may find that allowing your knees to bend a little will help to flatten your back—keep your bottom well lifted. When you have rested down allow yourself a moment to reflect on the space you appear to have created in your body.

2. Inhale as you lift first onto knees, then push into the inverted V of the Dog. Try to take the heels as far to the floor as possible, at the same time pushing the bottom up - this will help to straighten and flatten the back. Pull the abdomen back. Feel your shoulders widen but your back flatten. Your neck is long and ears kept between inner arms. Breathe easily. When you are ready, lower down onto the knees and then down into your starting position. Repeat twice.

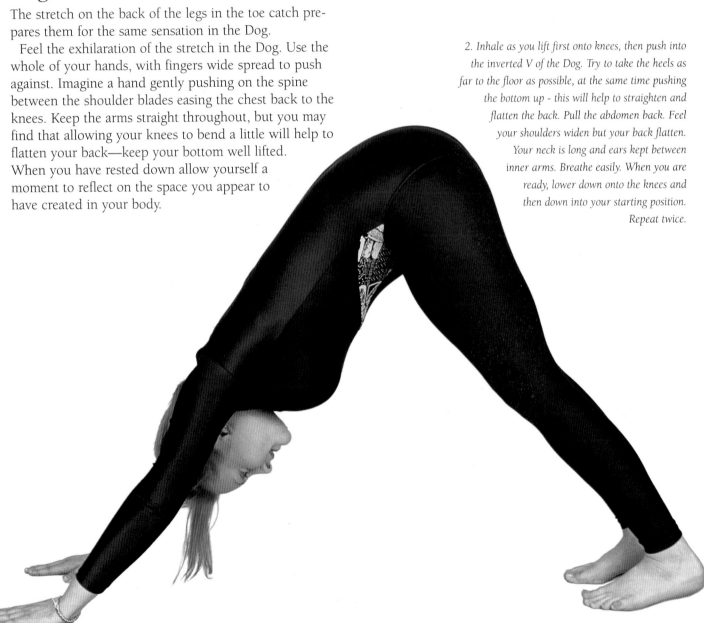

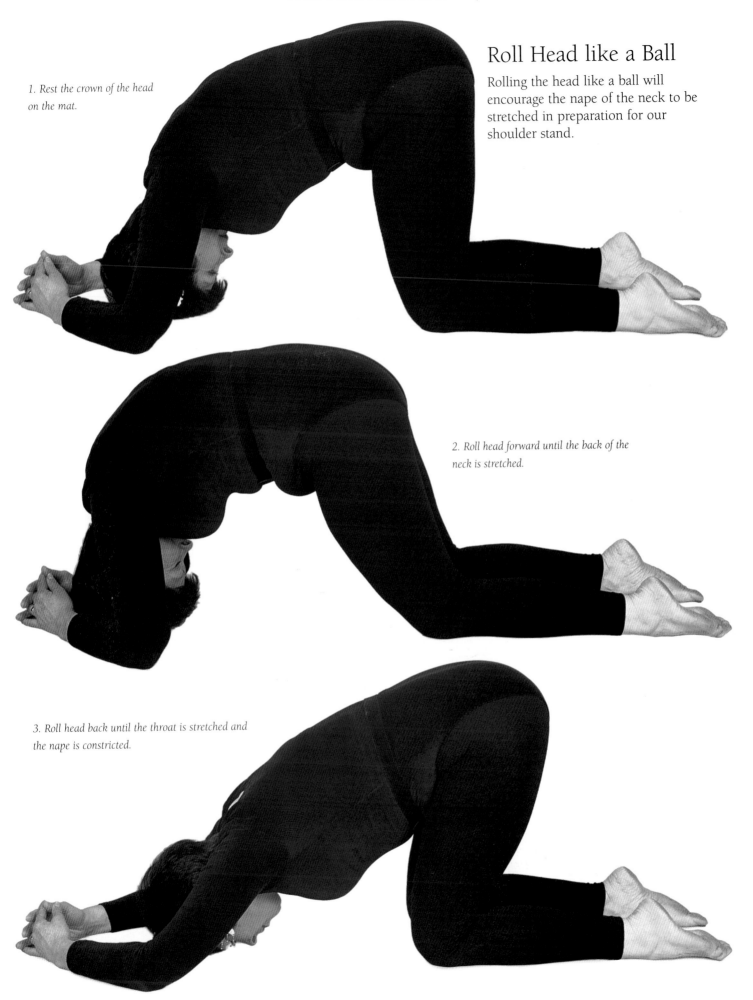

Roll Head like a Ball

Rolling the head like a ball will encourage the nape of the neck to be stretched in preparation for our shoulder stand.

1. Rest the crown of the head on the mat.

2. Roll head forward until the back of the neck is stretched.

3. Roll head back until the throat is stretched and the nape is constricted.

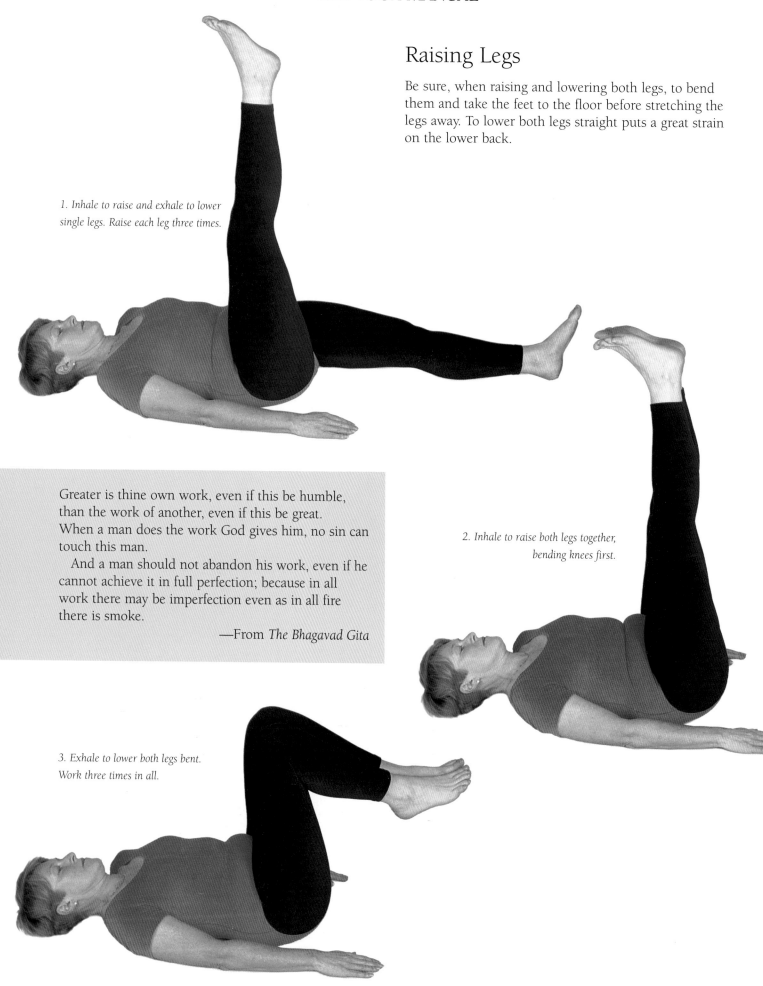

Raising Legs

Be sure, when raising and lowering both legs, to bend them and take the feet to the floor before stretching the legs away. To lower both legs straight puts a great strain on the lower back.

1. Inhale to raise and exhale to lower single legs. Raise each leg three times.

Greater is thine own work, even if this be humble, than the work of another, even if this be great. When a man does the work God gives him, no sin can touch this man.

And a man should not abandon his work, even if he cannot achieve it in full perfection; because in all work there may be imperfection even as in all fire there is smoke.

—From *The Bhagavad Gita*

2. Inhale to raise both legs together, bending knees first.

3. Exhale to lower both legs bent. Work three times in all.

Paripurna Navasana: Boat Posture

The Boat Posture asks us to work hard on the abdominal muscles. Hold the posture if you want to but breathe normally. You will discover the work on the abdomen! Try and come down with control—let the heels and shoulders touch the mat at the same time. Relax and allow the stomach muscles to soften.

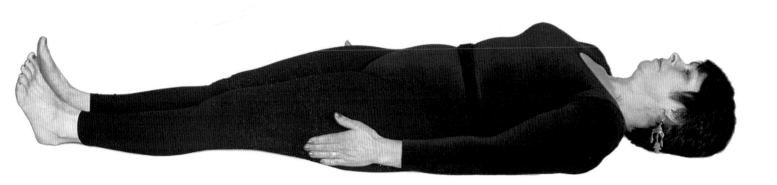

Lie flat with palms resting on sides of thighs.

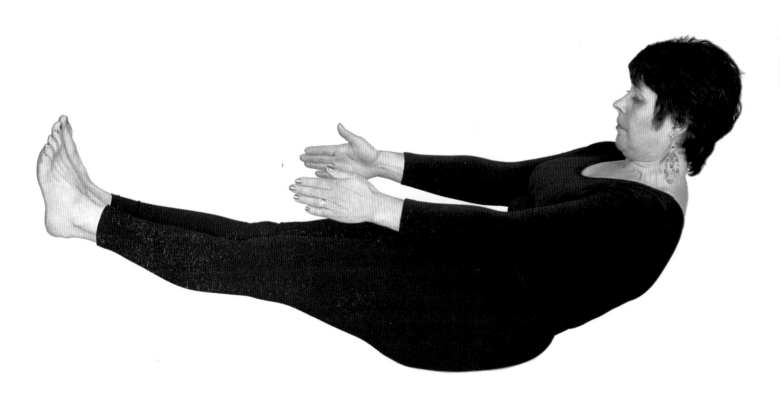

Inhale and lift legs and upper back—not too high—with arms outstretched. Endeavor to take eyes and toes to the same height.

Paripurna Navasana: Boat Posture II

An alternative version of this posture is attempted from a sitting position.

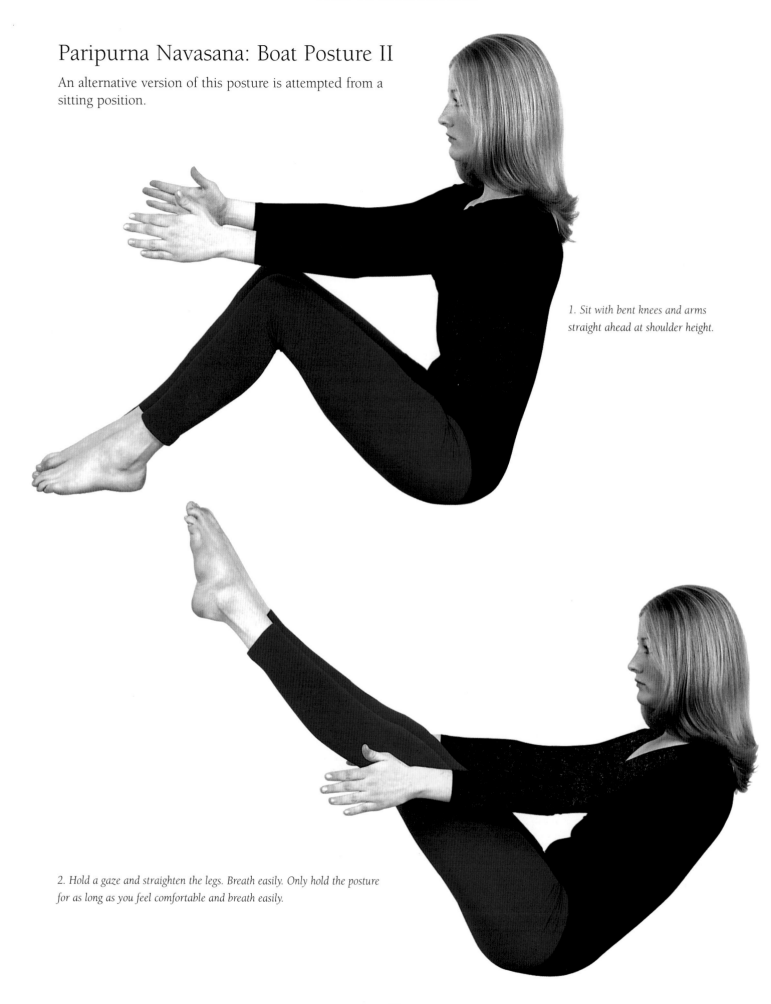

1. Sit with bent knees and arms straight ahead at shoulder height.

2. Hold a gaze and straighten the legs. Breath easily. Only hold the posture for as long as you feel comfortable and breath easily.

Sarvangasana: Shoulder Stand

Work slowly through the first modified stages of the shoulder stand and get used to them before you attempt the full posture. You may simply enjoy the ease on tired legs, and those with varicose veins, as you let them rest up the wall, or even fall apart as they lie upwards but supported.

If you enjoyed the shoulder stand, you may like to attempt the plough.

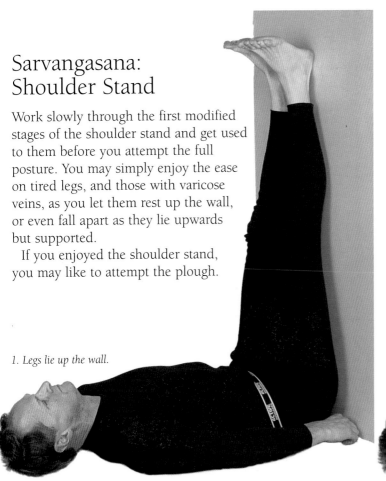

1. Legs lie up the wall.

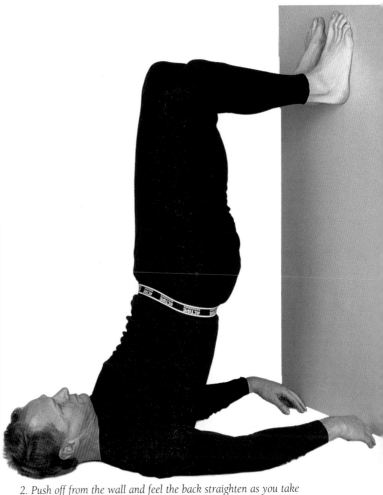

2. Push off from the wall and feel the back straighten as you take the chest towards the chin.

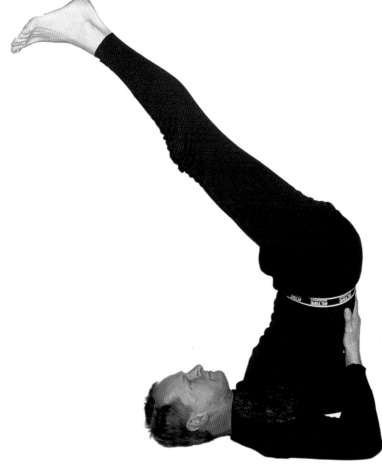

3. Lie flat and simply lift the legs and push the back off the floor. Immediately support the back with the hands. This is a modified version of shoulder stand called candle pose.

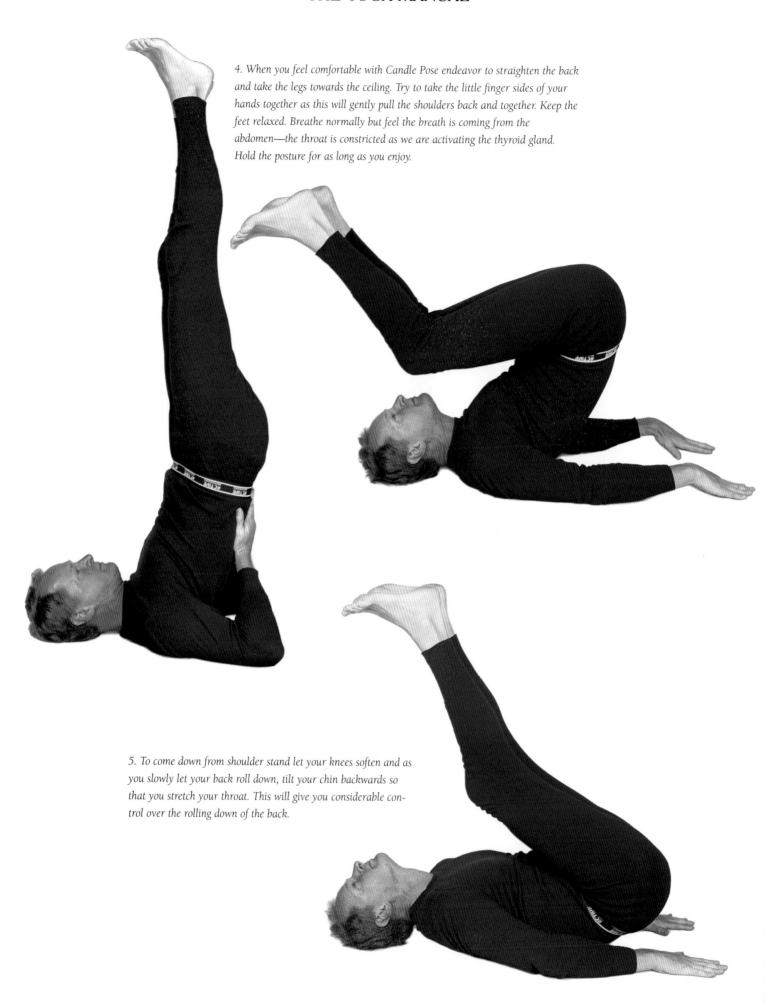

4. When you feel comfortable with Candle Pose endeavor to straighten the back and take the legs towards the ceiling. Try to take the little finger sides of your hands together as this will gently pull the shoulders back and together. Keep the feet relaxed. Breathe normally but feel the breath is coming from the abdomen—the throat is constricted as we are activating the thyroid gland. Hold the posture for as long as you enjoy.

5. To come down from shoulder stand let your knees soften and as you slowly let your back roll down, tilt your chin backwards so that you stretch your throat. This will give you considerable control over the rolling down of the back.

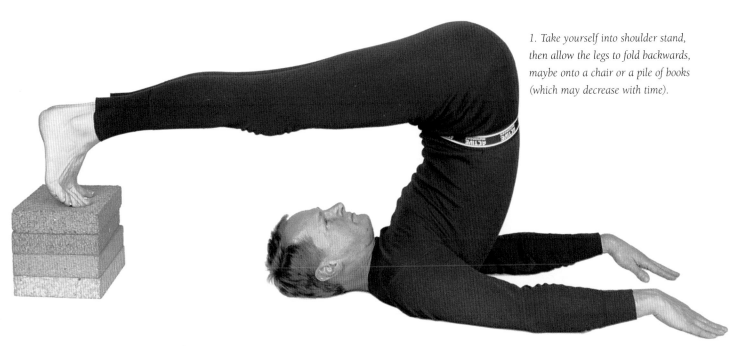

1. Take yourself into shoulder stand, then allow the legs to fold backwards, maybe onto a chair or a pile of books (which may decrease with time).

Halasana: Plough Posture

When in the plough feel the back is straight and lifted. The plough stretches the whole of the back of the body, and the next posture will compensate for this. You will feel a constriction in the nape of the neck and the upper back (which has recently been stretched) and a stretch in the throat and down the chest.

2. Eventually, you may feel you can take your feet to the floor. Turn your toes under and aim your heels towards the floor. Link the fingers and stretch them away to ease back the shoulders. Your buttocks stretch to the ceiling and your chest is close to your chin. Breathe comfortably directing your breath in and out of your abdomen but if there is any strain come out of the posture. Hold the posture for a short time initially, and roll out of it in the same way as the shoulder stand by tilting the chin.

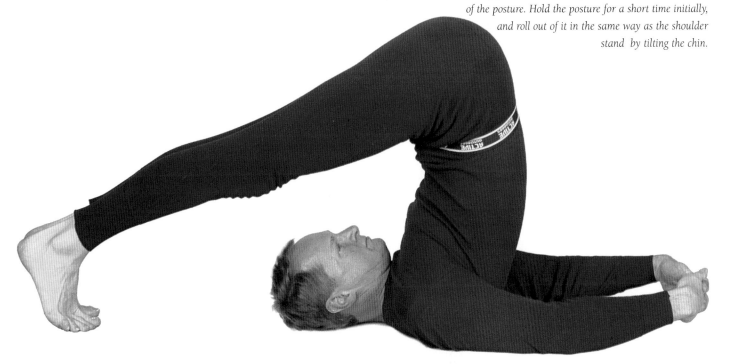

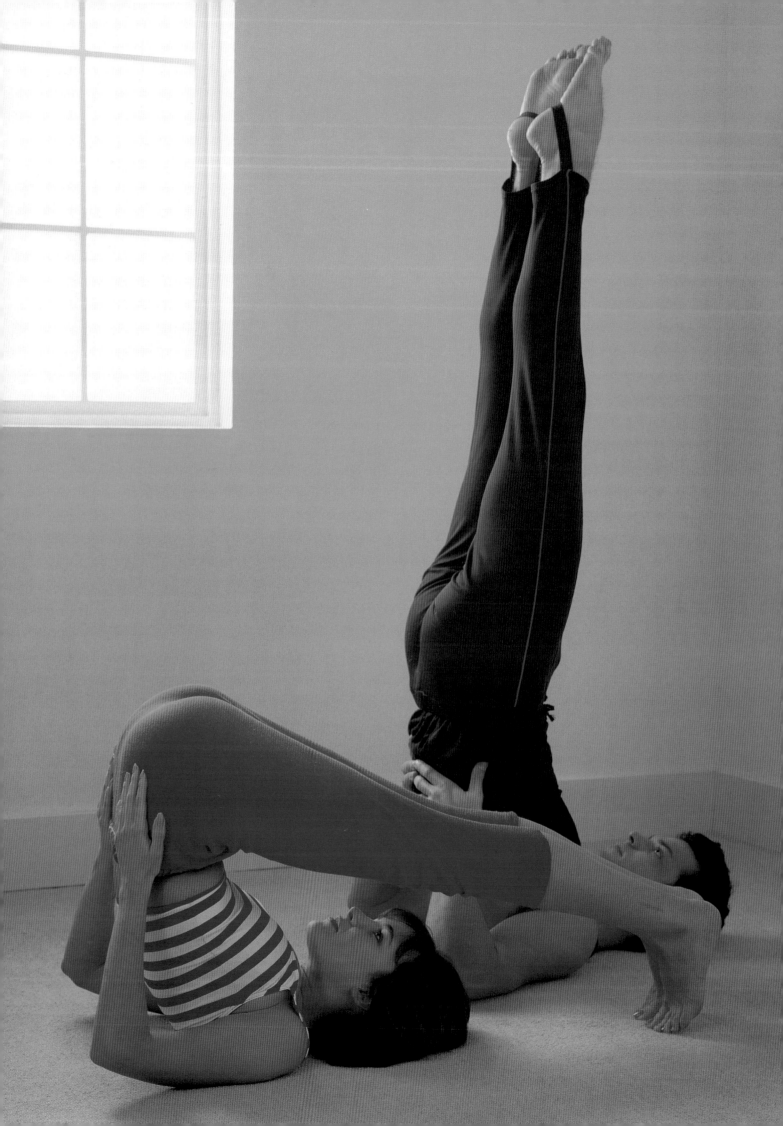

Opposite: Shoulder Stand and Plough

Open Chest Drop

This posture will compensate for the Shoulder Stand and Plough by relaxing the back instead of lifting it.

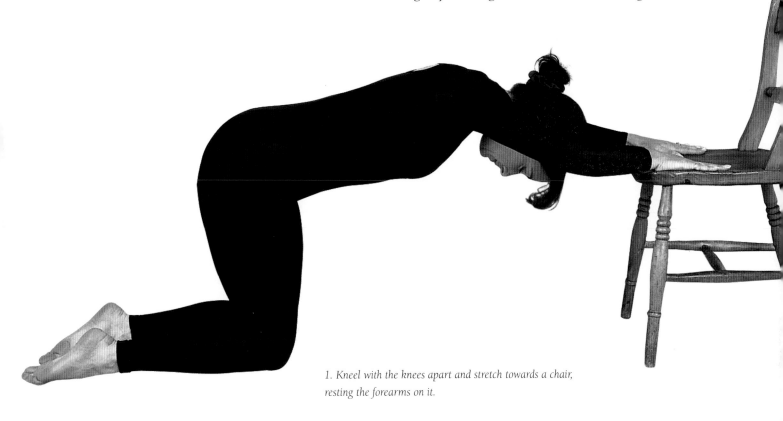

1. Kneel with the knees apart and stretch towards a chair, resting the forearms on it.

2. Allow the back to sink down and the bottom to push away. Keep the head in line with the spine and the back neck long. Feel the work on the shoulders. Breathe normally and hold for as long as is comfortable.

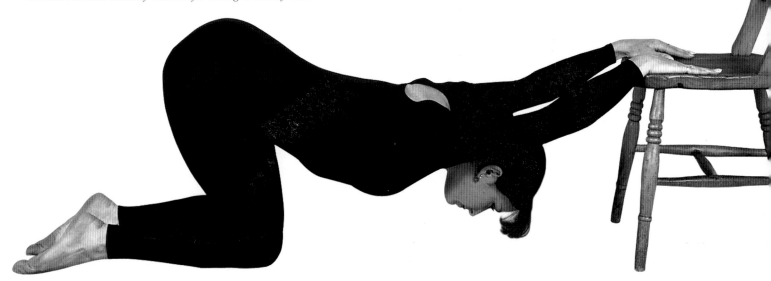

Modified Half-Spinal Twist

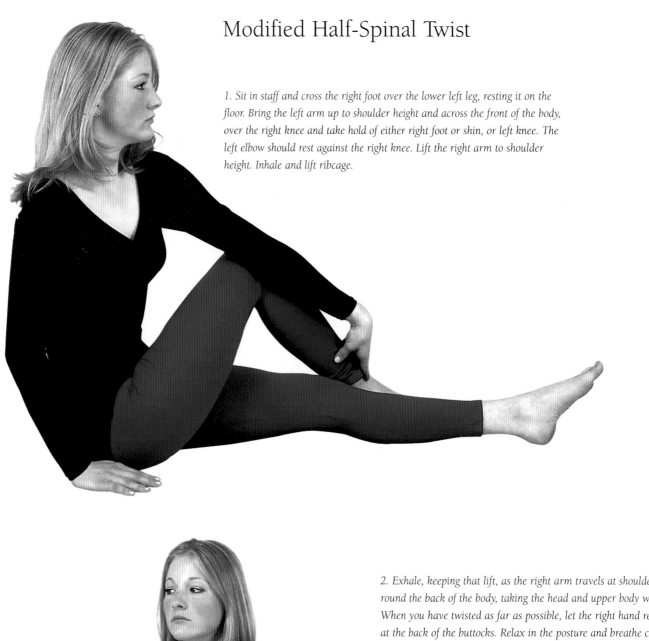

1. Sit in staff and cross the right foot over the lower left leg, resting it on the floor. Bring the left arm up to shoulder height and across the front of the body, over the right knee and take hold of either right foot or shin, or left knee. The left elbow should rest against the right knee. Lift the right arm to shoulder height. Inhale and lift ribcage.

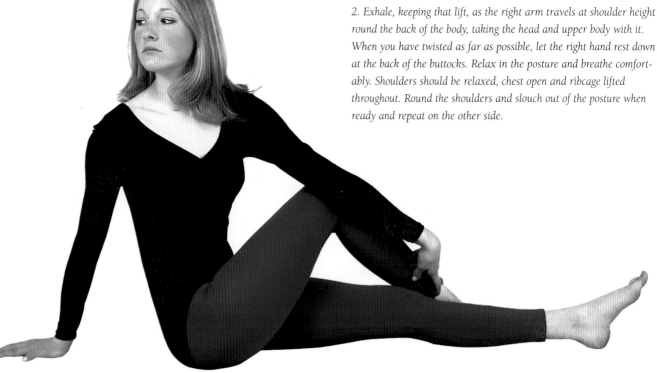

2. Exhale, keeping that lift, as the right arm travels at shoulder height round the back of the body, taking the head and upper body with it. When you have twisted as far as possible, let the right hand rest down at the back of the buttocks. Relax in the posture and breathe comfortably. Shoulders should be relaxed, chest open and ribcage lifted throughout. Round the shoulders and slouch out of the posture when ready and repeat on the other side.

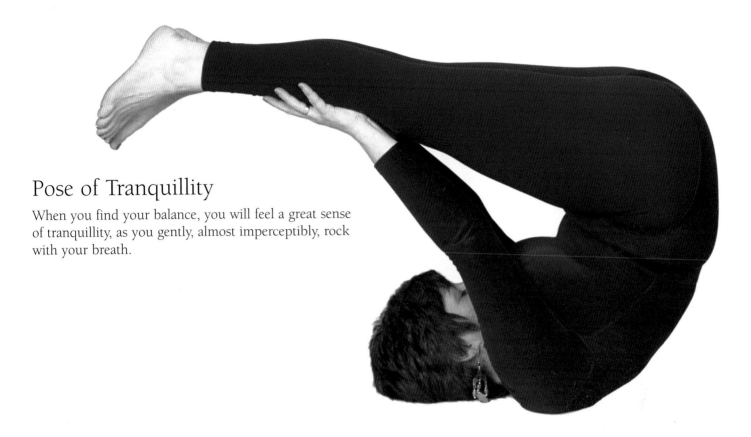

Pose of Tranquillity

When you find your balance, you will feel a great sense of tranquillity, as you gently, almost imperceptibly, rock with your breath.

Lift into Candle Pose then take the hands to rest just below the knees. Elbows must be straight and the whole weight of the legs resting on the palms. This is a balance and you may need to experiment.

Tadasana: Mountain Posture

Standing relaxation. Feet parallel, pelvis level, ribcage lifted, head erect and shoulders relaxed.

If you are content, close your eyes, otherwise allow your gaze to fall to the floor. When you feel quite comfortable and your breath is even, begin to visualize a tree—a big mature tree of your choice. See yourself as this tree. As you inhale, see your tree grow a fraction taller, and as you exhale feel its roots grow a little deeper into the earth. Enjoy the feeling of strength, power, increased stability and reliability you gain from this visualization.

When ready allow the breath to deepen and open your eyes. You will feel your feet are particularly reluctant to break their roots and lift. Be sure to feel totally re-orientated before moving around.

HAPPINESS

So they all ran about looking for Happiness, calling "Happiness, Happiness, where are you?" And every so often they found some. And they would hold it for a moment and smile and exclaim, "I've got some!" But they were so used to looking for it that after a while they would start running about again, automatically calling, "Happiness, Happiness, where are you?" dropping their happiness on the ground and trampling it underfoot as they ran.

—Susan Palmer-Jones

CHAPTER FIVE
BACKWARD BENDS

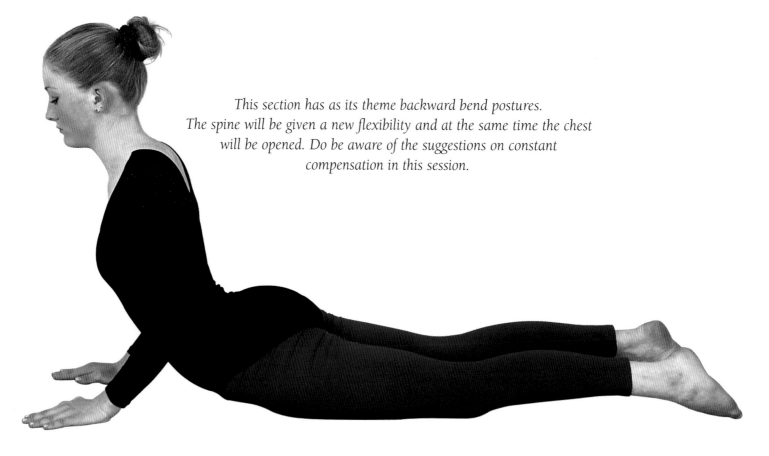

*This section has as its theme backward bend postures.
The spine will be given a new flexibility and at the same time the chest
will be opened. Do be aware of the suggestions on constant
compensation in this session.*

Go placidly amid the noise and haste and remember
what peace there may be in silence.
—From the *Desiderata*

Relax in Savasana. Yield to the mat. This quieting of the senses to begin is as important as the postures.

When you feel calm and comfortable, bring your awareness to the spine. In Yoga, we see the exhalation breath as golden and warm, so with each out breath feel that warmth flow down the spine. Let it become soft, pliable and warm.

After these few moments, allow your attention to leave the spine, your breath to return to normal.

Stretch and Curl

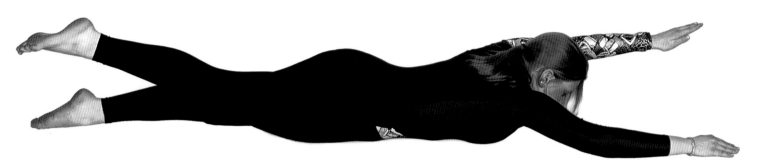

Lifting Arms and Legs

Be aware of how your back feels in this posture. There may not be a great deal of movement, but this is a strong posture. Bring arms to the sides and relax. Compensate for that strong backward bend with a rounding of the back.

1. Lie flat on your front with arms outstretched along the floor. Inhale and raise a diagonal arm and leg. Do not look along your arm—raise your head alongside your arm, but keep eyes downcast, so the back of the neck is long. Exhale as you lower. Work twice on each diagonal.

2. Inhale and lift all four limbs. Again raise your head alongside your arms but do not lift your eyes. Exhale to lower. Repeat once.

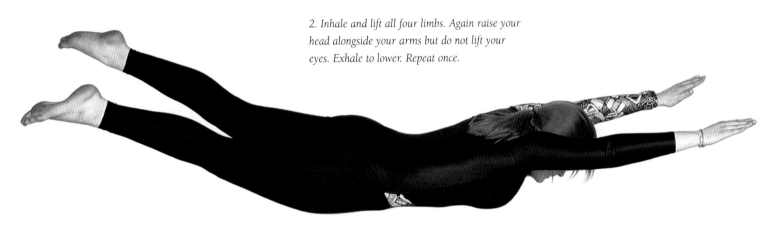

Perfect peace
Does not exist.
Everywhere there is
The hum of life,
The noise of the city,
The call of the wild.
Silence does not exist
Because life is not silent.
Peace comes from within.
In each and everyone of us
There is a still quiet place
Deep inside.
—Maria Garner

Pindasana: Pose of a Child

If it is not possible or easy to take the head all the way to the floor in the pose of a child, bring the arms round and let the head rest on loosely-made fists. Try to keep your bottom resting down on your feet.

Sit back on heels and take the head to the floor until the hairline rests. Arms rest on the floor with hands by the feet, so shoulders fall forward and back rounds. Breathe easily.

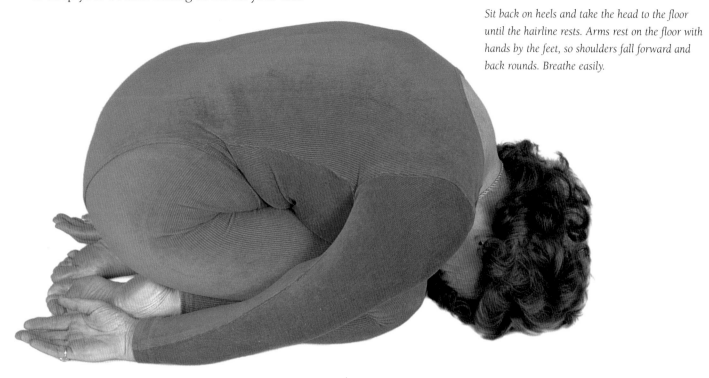

Exhale as you bring a knee towards your face.
Inhale as you stretch that leg away along with the opposite arm. Keep the eyes cast down and back neck long. Repeat twice on this diagonal and work three times on the other.

Cat with Arms and Legs

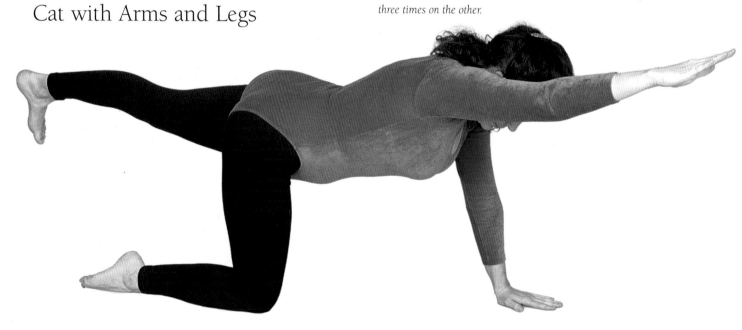

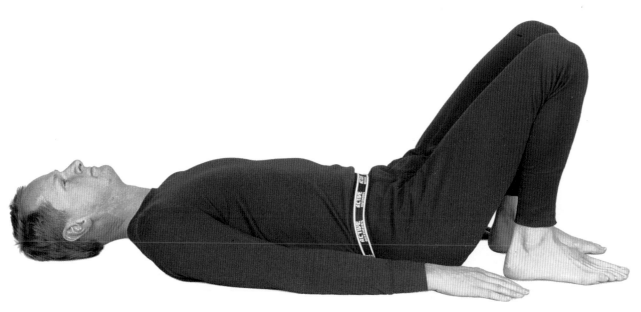

Dvipada Pitham: Hip Raise

You may enjoy the visualization of your spine as a string of pearls, each vertebra is a pearl and moves independently. In this way, you will achieve a rolling.

1. Lie with knees crooked and parallel feet close in to the buttocks at the hip width apart. Keep the back of the neck long and allow arms to rest by the sides.

2. Begin with lifting the bottom, raise the back off the floor until you feel you take the weight up onto the shoulders. The chest is aimed towards the ceiling. Lower in the same way, being sure to feel the roll of the back up and down rather than simply a lift and lower. Repeat twice then hug the knees to the chest to compensate.

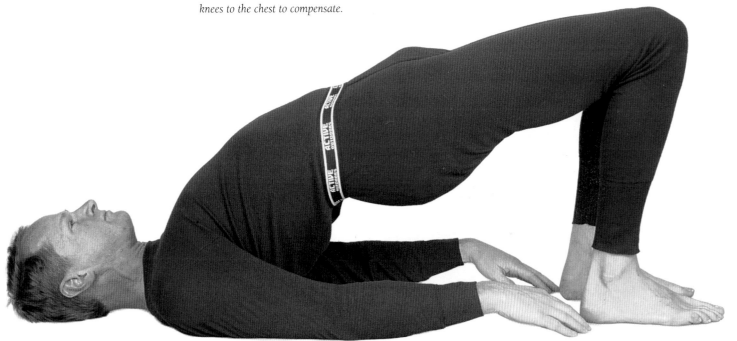

Bhujangasana: Cobra

You will have felt the constriction in the waist and kidney area of the back. As this constriction is released with the relaxation, so fresh blood can flow into the kidneys and cleanse them. The posture activates the bladder and flushes out stored toxins.

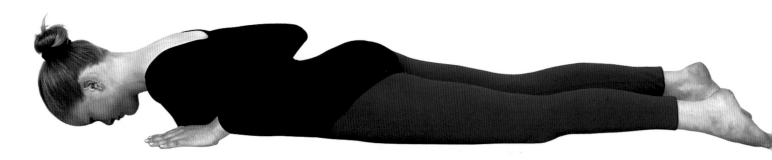

1. Rest down with forehead on the mat and hands under shoulders. The elbows are neatly tucked in and remain so. Tuck the tail under and so feel the spine lengthen before you begin.

2. Inhale and lift until the upper body is off the mat, but the navel remains close to the mat, so elbows stay bent. Lift and lengthen the neck, and drop the hips. Relax the legs and feet. Breathe normally in the posture. Exhale as you relax down. Turn the cheek and allow the arms to rest by the sides, so shoulders fall into the floor. Relax. Repeat twice more. After a period of relaxation and reflection push up into the Pose of a Child.

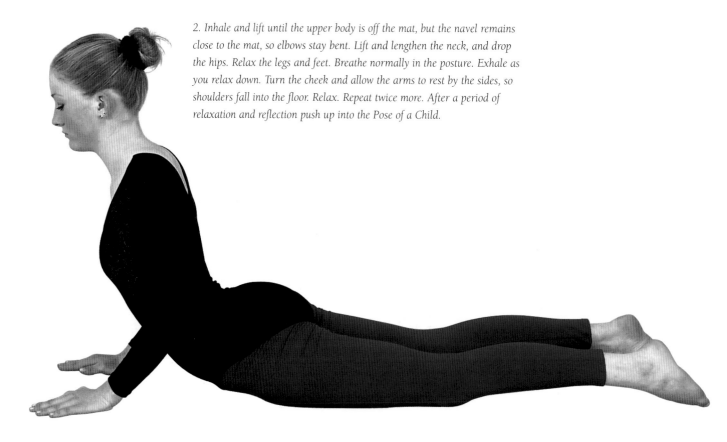

Salabhasana: Locust

In the locust the constriction will be felt lower down the
back, below the waist. If you feel able to hold the posture
do not hold your breath.

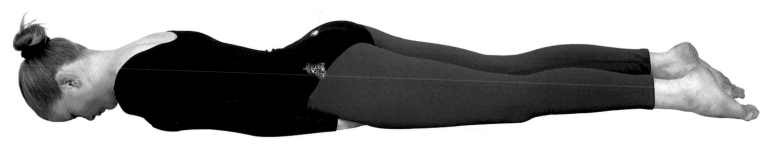

Make fists and take them into the groin to lie along straight arms. Rest the
forehead on the mat and endeavor to keep it there throughout. Inhale.

Exhale and lift the body from the waist down. Again this posture is strong
so initially you may not want to hold it at all. Relax down as you inhale
and repeat twice. Relax into the Pose of a Child to round the back.

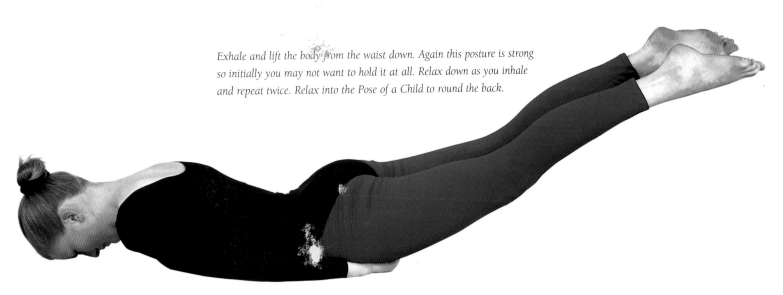

Dhanurasana: Bow

The bow posture is a combination of the two previous ones. We can take advantage of the arching of the back for a very strong posture, the camel.

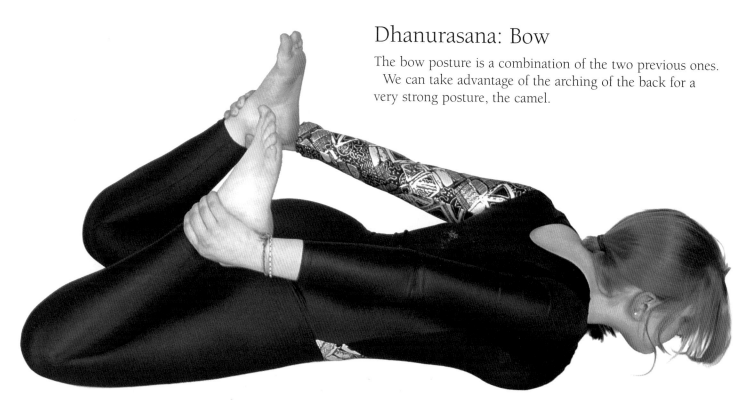

1. Begin by lying face down, bending up knees, and taking hold of feet or ankles. Inhale.

2. Exhale and attempt to lift head and shoulders and thighs from the floor. Allow the legs and feet to feel uplifted and the arms and shoulders to be directing them forward towards the raised head. Breathe easily and feel a gentle abdominal rock. Hold for as long as is comfortable.

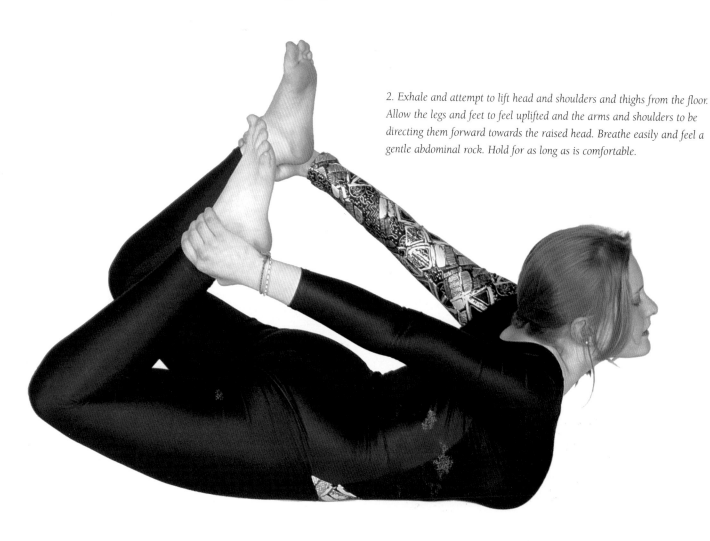

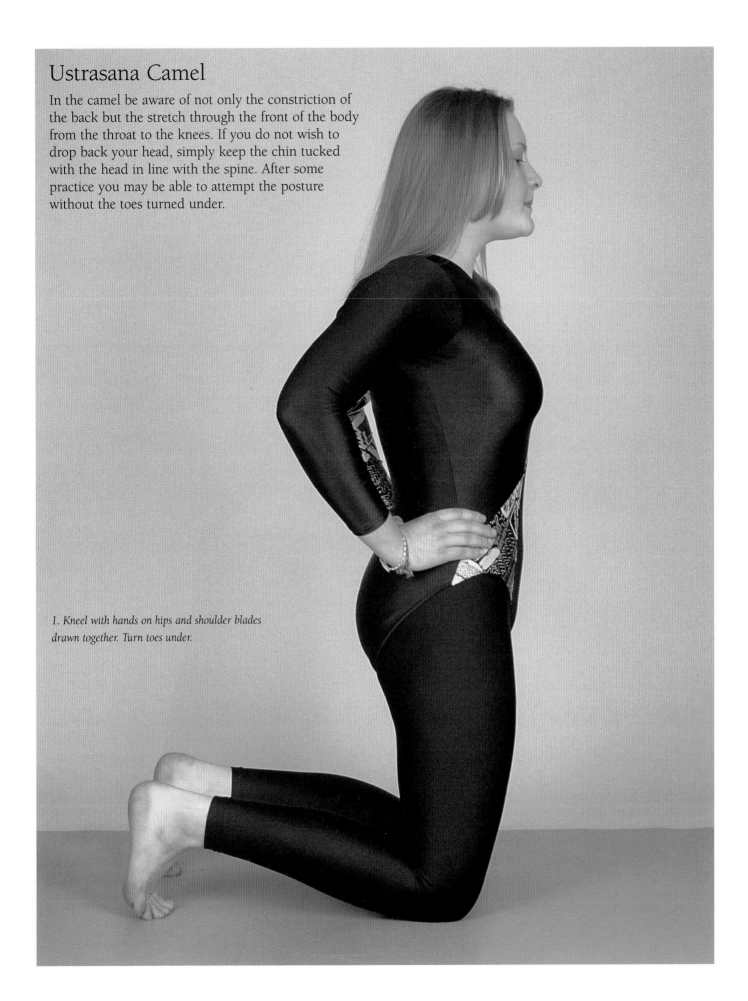

Ustrasana Camel

In the camel be aware of not only the constriction of the back but the stretch through the front of the body from the throat to the knees. If you do not wish to drop back your head, simply keep the chin tucked with the head in line with the spine. After some practice you may be able to attempt the posture without the toes turned under.

1. Kneel with hands on hips and shoulder blades drawn together. Turn toes under.

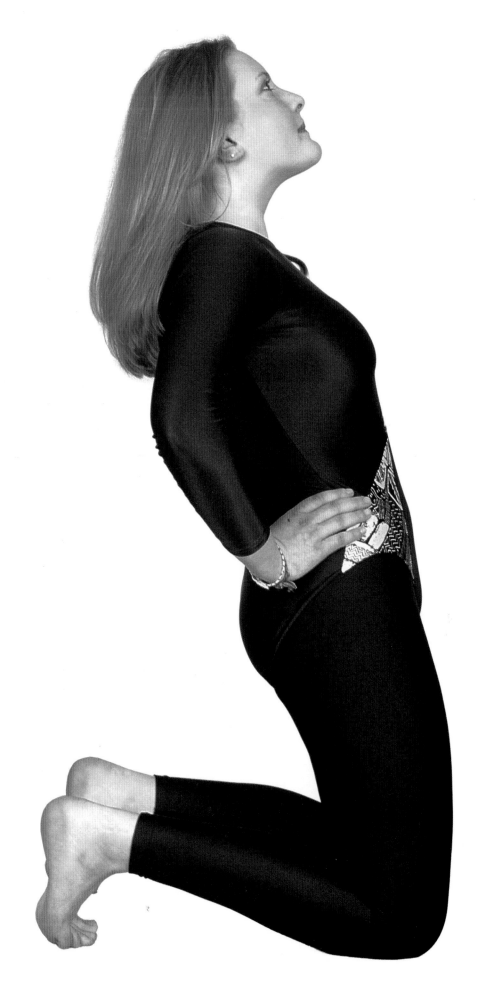

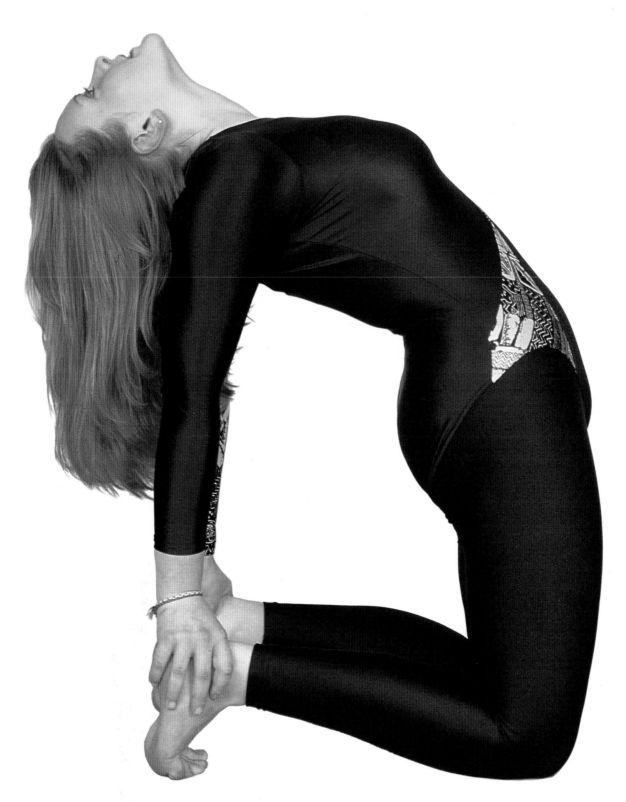

As you exhale, the upper body is allowed to lean back, very carefully dropping the head backwards and allowing the hands to reach back to grasp the heels. Take the chest towards the ceiling and thighs to ninety degrees to the floor. Breathe normally. Lift out of the posture, raising the head very carefully on an inhalation and immediately roll down into the Pose of a Child. Repeat twice if you are happy to do so.

These last two postures are very strong. Only attempt them with care and if it is comfortable to do so.

Ardha Matsyendrasana: The Spinal Twist

Natarajasana: The Dancer

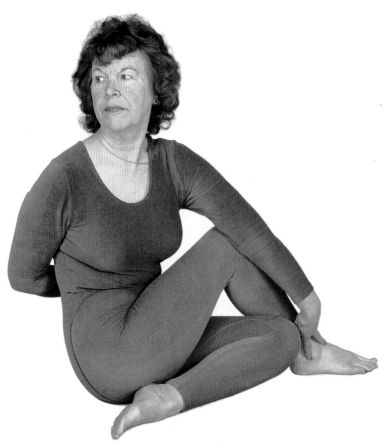

Sit in Dandasana. Bend the left knee and take the foot under the right leg to rest by the right buttock. Bend the right knee to rest the foot on the floor just in front of the left knee. Turn the body towards the right and bring the left arm over the right knee to hold the right foot. Breathe in and lift the ribcage. Exhale and take the right arm round to the back, taking the upper body with it. Let that arm rest in the small of the back. Hold the posture with open chest, relaxed shoulders and comfortable breath. Slouch out of it when ready, unwind and repeat on the other side. Relax in the corpse position for a while.

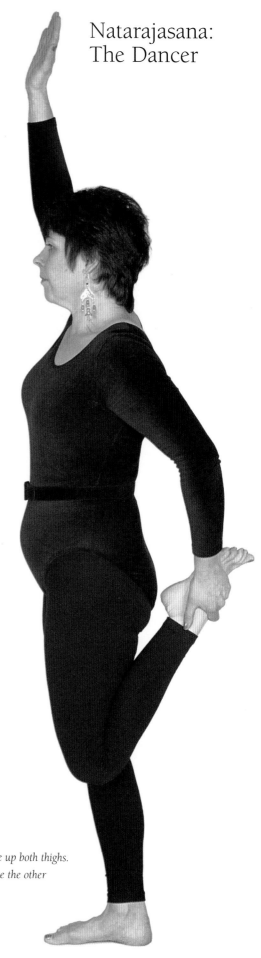

1. Stand tall, bend a knee and grasp the foot. Try to line up both thighs. Let the gaze fall down to the floor close to the body. Take the other hand overhead and stretch tall as you inhale.

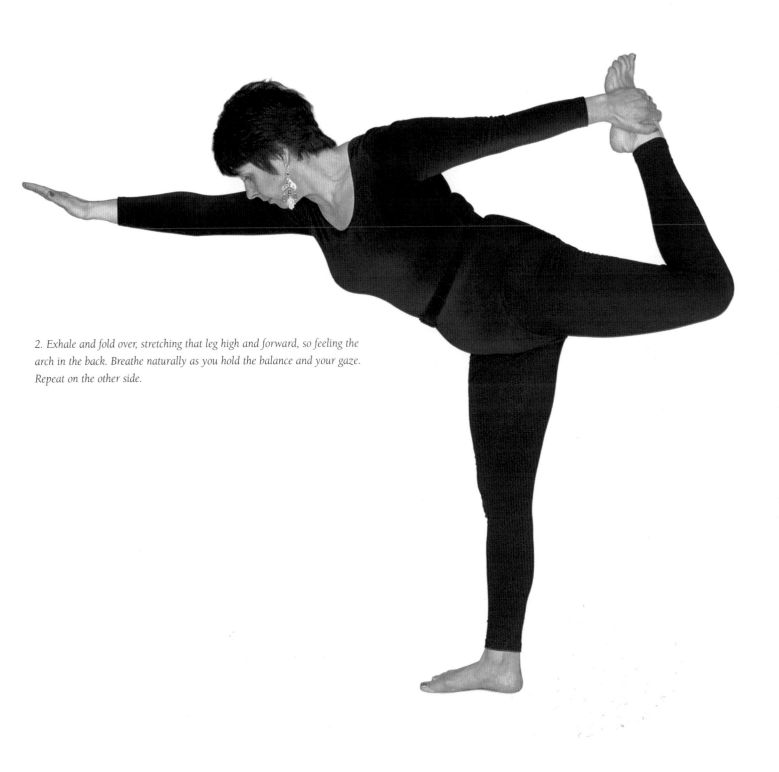

2. Exhale and fold over, stretching that leg high and forward, so feeling the arch in the back. Breathe naturally as you hold the balance and your gaze. Repeat on the other side.

Nadi Shodhan: Pranayama
Alternate Nostril Breath

The alternate nostril breath gives great tranquillity as it gently massages the pituitary gland at the bottom of the brain.

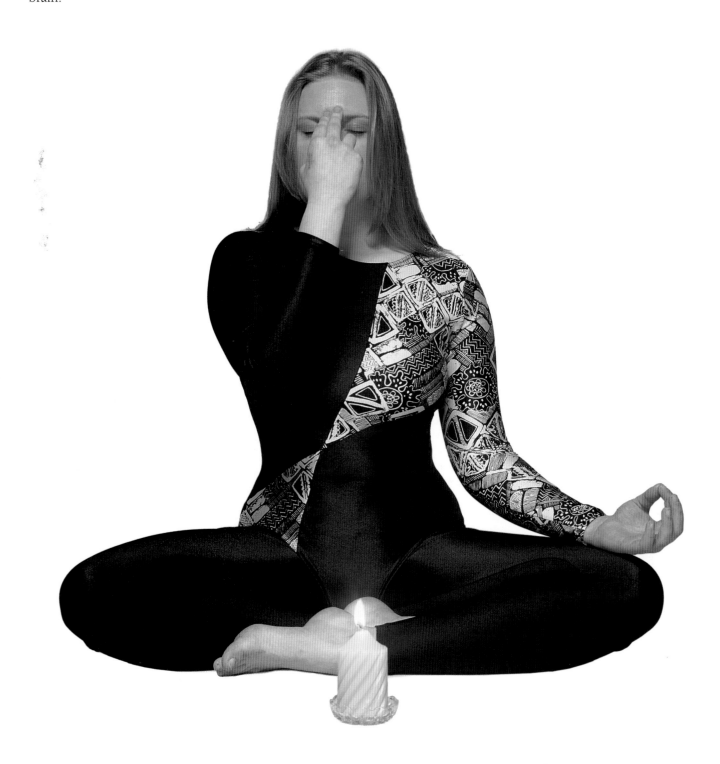

Yoga Nidra: Total Relaxation

Relax and sink into the mat. Be aware that this Yoga session has asked you to be brave—there is both a physical and psychological exposure as the back is arched and the chest opened.

As you relax, your breath is calm and your thoughts drifting, think through your whole body allowing it to relax and soften. Be conscious now of your solar plexus and see a golden sun resting there. With each inhalation the warmth and glow from that sun is replenished.

When that sun begins to fade, hold onto the glow, the energy you have acquired. Deepen your breath, stretch, and yawn before rolling over onto your right side, opening your eyes and sitting up.

Arise out of yourself,
Let go the garment of the body:
Seek the place of healing and silence and tranquillity,
Seek the lake of peace within,
Calm and tideless.
Let the boat of the mind glide slowly from its moorings
(Leave the turbulent, restless river)
Past the soft green fingers of the rushes,
Into the lake's cool silver,
Quiet rippling at the prow.
There is calm here and awareness of nature,
So be tranquil and aware of God.
—From a poem by Teddy Dent

Opposite: Sit comfortably in easy pose, half-lotus or full lotus with spine straight and head erect. When your breath feels comfortable and your body relaxed, take the right hand to the face and place the index finger and middle finger on the third eye between the eyebrows, the ring finger to rest by the left nostril and the thumb to rest by the right. Close off the right nostril with the thumb and inhale through the left. Close off the left nostril, open the right and exhale through it. Inhale back through the right, then close it off and exhale through the left. Continue in this way, exhaling and inhaling back through the same nostril. Slow and lengthen the breath as much as possible and be aware of that instant of pause at the end of each inhalation before the body needs to exhale.

CHAPTER SIX
A LITTLE HARDER

*This section consists of more advanced postures and, if you are new to Yoga,
you should work through the other sections before attempting them.*

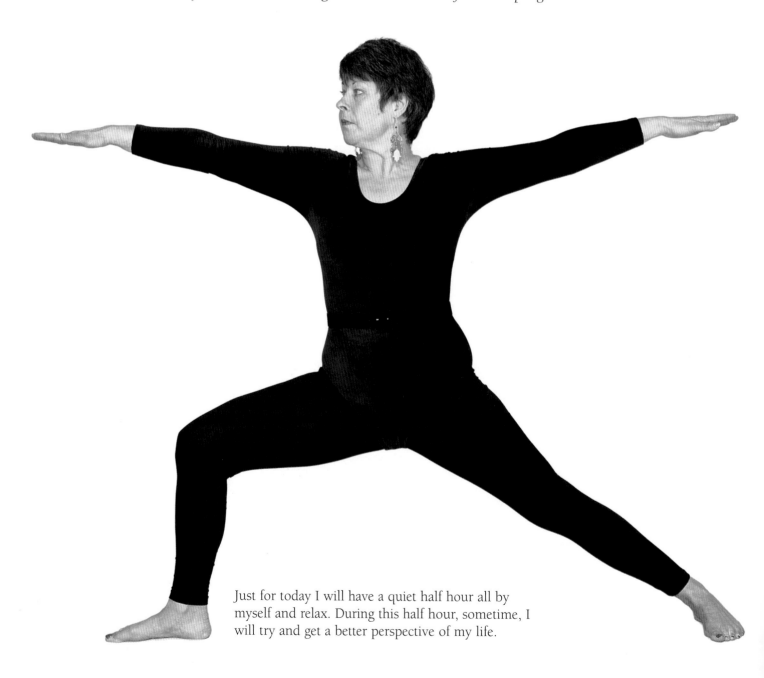

Just for today I will have a quiet half hour all by
myself and relax. During this half hour, sometime, I
will try and get a better perspective of my life.

Begin in Savasana. Check through the body, directing the breath into the whole of the body—concentration on this exercise of directing the breath will tend to bring your total awareness onto your Yoga and enable you to temporarily cut off from the stresses of life. When you return to any stressful situations, as doubtless you will from time to time, you will be refreshed and more clear-minded to deal with them.

Pranayama: Calming Breath

By making the exhalation breath last longer than the inhalation we can calm ourselves. A way to achieve this is to count as you breath, for example counting up to eight as you inhale and up to twelve as you exhale. If these numbers do not fit your breath rhythm, then make up your own—simply make the out count longer than the in. After perhaps seven calming breaths, allow the breath to return to normal. When ready, stretch and curl.

Look well to this day
For it is life,
The very best of life.
In its brief course lie all
The realities and truths of existence—
The joy of growth,
The splendour of action,
The glory of power.
For yesterday is but a memory,
And tomorrow only a vision,
But today, if well-lived, makes
Every yesterday a memory of happiness
And every tomorrow a vision of hope.
Look well, therefore, to this day.
—Sanskrit Poem

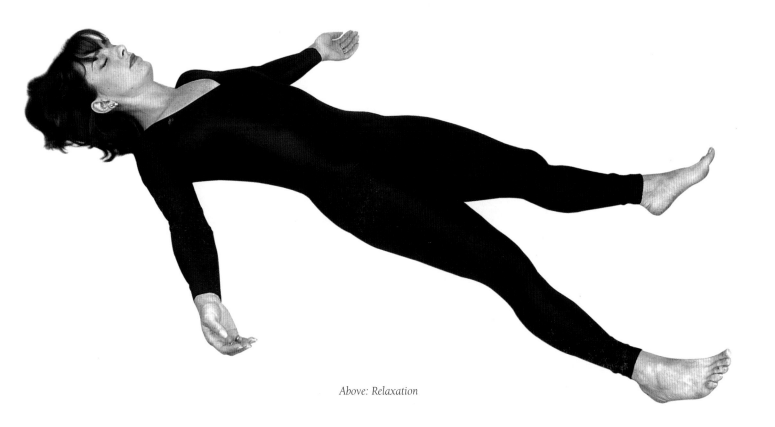

Above: Relaxation

Hamstring Stretch

To stretch the hamstring, the muscle at the back of the leg, it is necessary to keep the leg straight. It is better to move just an inch towards the face in this way rather than a long way with a bent knee.

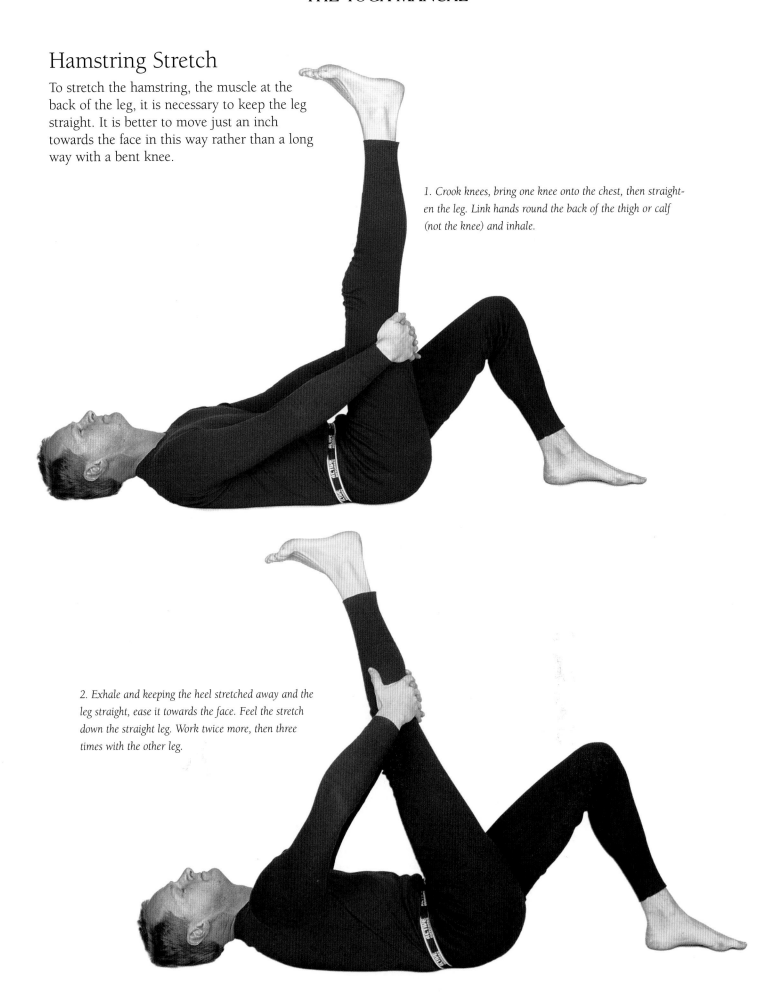

1. Crook knees, bring one knee onto the chest, then straighten the leg. Link hands round the back of the thigh or calf (not the knee) and inhale.

2. Exhale and keeping the heel stretched away and the leg straight, ease it towards the face. Feel the stretch down the straight leg. Work twice more, then three times with the other leg.

Inner Thigh Stretch

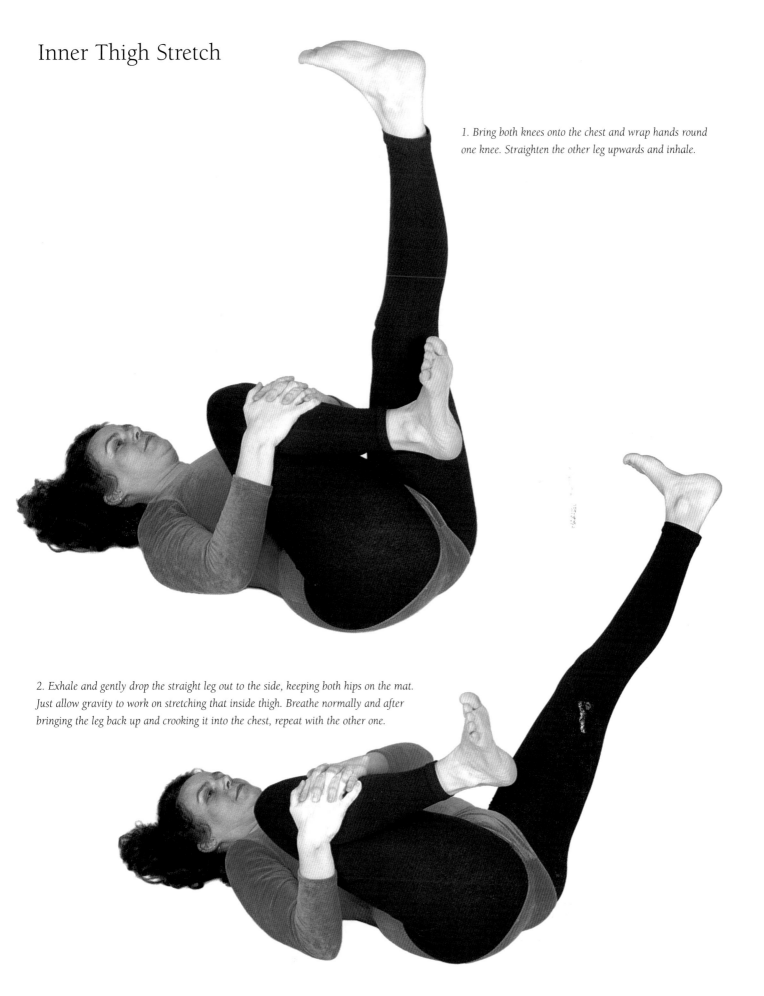

1. Bring both knees onto the chest and wrap hands round one knee. Straighten the other leg upwards and inhale.

2. Exhale and gently drop the straight leg out to the side, keeping both hips on the mat. Just allow gravity to work on stretching that inside thigh. Breathe normally and after bringing the leg back up and crooking it into the chest, repeat with the other one.

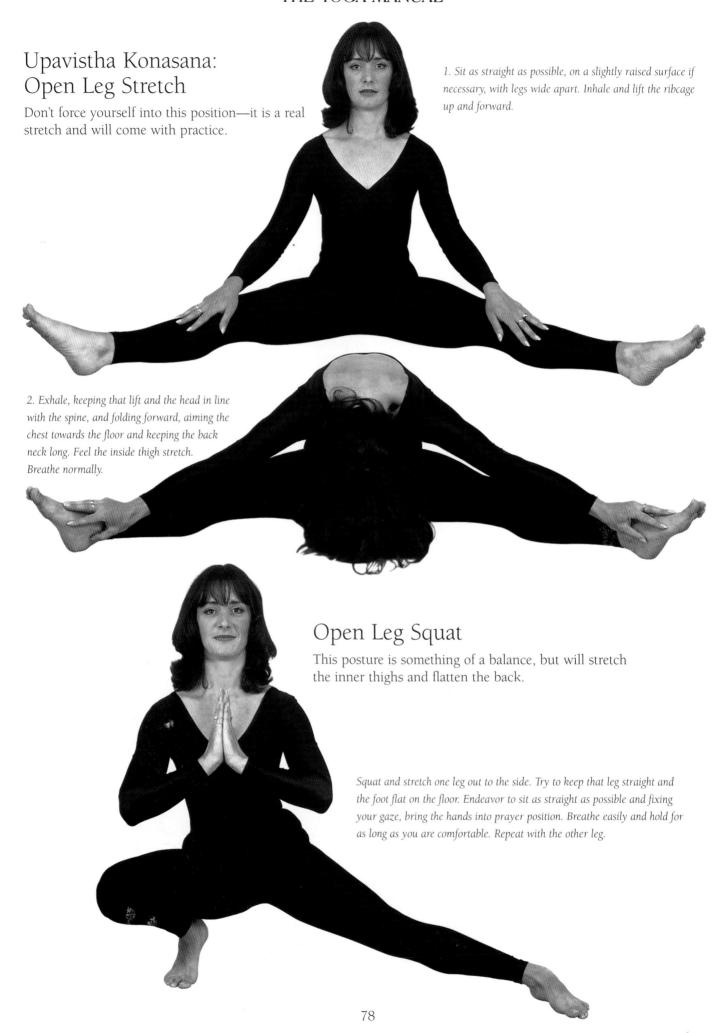

Upavistha Konasana: Open Leg Stretch

Don't force yourself into this position—it is a real stretch and will come with practice.

1. Sit as straight as possible, on a slightly raised surface if necessary, with legs wide apart. Inhale and lift the ribcage up and forward.

2. Exhale, keeping that lift and the head in line with the spine, and folding forward, aiming the chest towards the floor and keeping the back neck long. Feel the inside thigh stretch. Breathe normally.

Open Leg Squat

This posture is something of a balance, but will stretch the inner thighs and flatten the back.

Squat and stretch one leg out to the side. Try to keep that leg straight and the foot flat on the floor. Endeavor to sit as straight as possible and fixing your gaze, bring the hands into prayer position. Breathe easily and hold for as long as you are comfortable. Repeat with the other leg.

Lunge

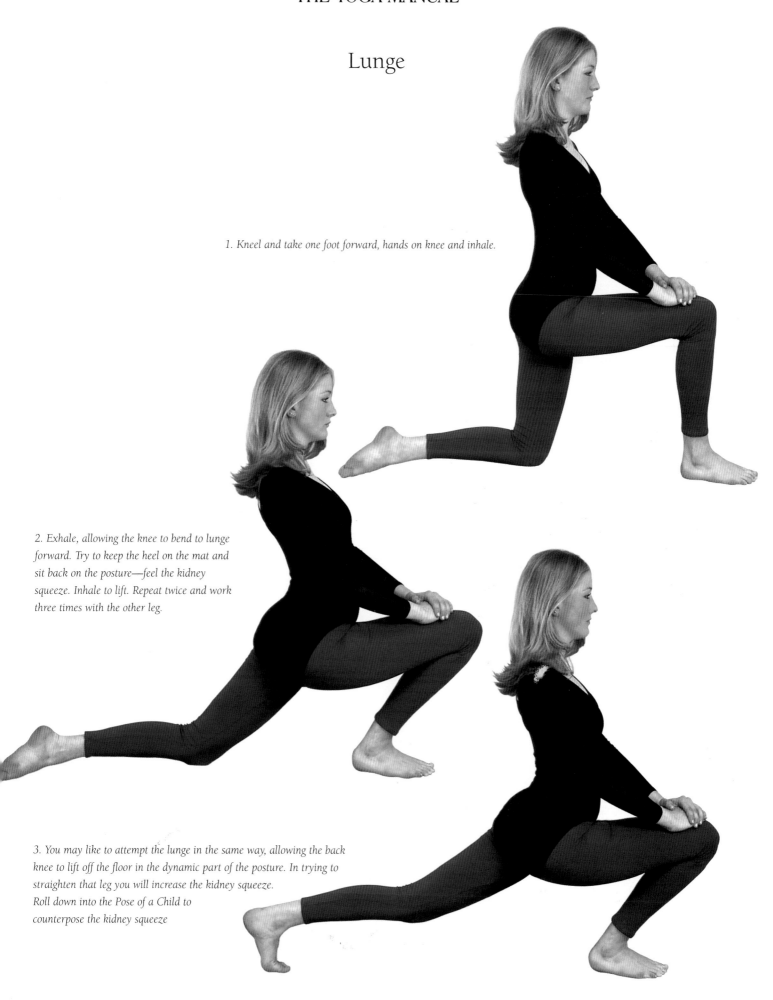

1. Kneel and take one foot forward, hands on knee and inhale.

2. Exhale, allowing the knee to bend to lunge forward. Try to keep the heel on the mat and sit back on the posture—feel the kidney squeeze. Inhale to lift. Repeat twice and work three times with the other leg.

3. You may like to attempt the lunge in the same way, allowing the back knee to lift off the floor in the dynamic part of the posture. In trying to straighten that leg you will increase the kidney squeeze. Roll down into the Pose of a Child to counterpose the kidney squeeze

Gomukhasana Head of a Cow

This posture will relax tension in the shoulders and neck. The constriction and then relaxation in the muscles at the side of the neck can help to prevent and ease headaches. It will perhaps be interesting to watch how differently the two sides of your body feel in the posture.

Uttanasana: Full Forward Bend with Flat Back

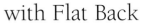

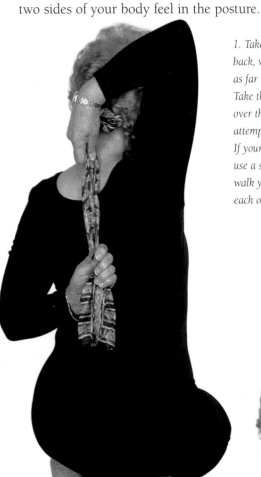

1. Take an arm up the back, wriggling the hand as far up as possible. Take the other arm back over the shoulder and attempt to link the fingers. If your hands do not meet, use a scarf or belt and walk your hands towards each other.

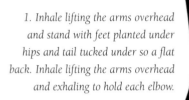

1. Inhale lifting the arms overhead and stand with feet planted under hips and tail tucked under so a flat back. Inhale lifting the arms overhead and exhaling to hold each elbow.

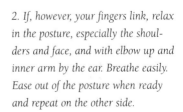

2. If, however, your fingers link, relax in the posture, especially the shoulders and face, and with elbow up and inner arm by the ear. Breathe easily. Ease out of the posture when ready and repeat on the other side.

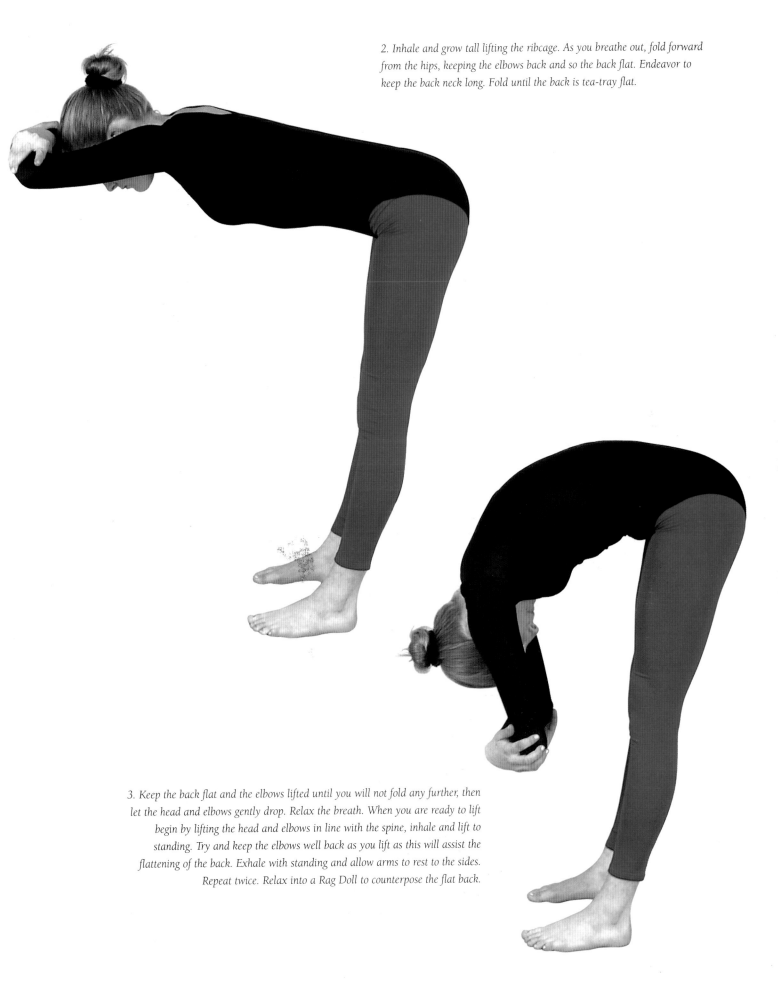

2. Inhale and grow tall lifting the ribcage. As you breathe out, fold forward from the hips, keeping the elbows back and so the back flat. Endeavor to keep the back neck long. Fold until the back is tea-tray flat.

3. Keep the back flat and the elbows lifted until you will not fold any further, then let the head and elbows gently drop. Relax the breath. When you are ready to lift begin by lifting the head and elbows in line with the spine, inhale and lift to standing. Try and keep the elbows well back as you lift as this will assist the flattening of the back. Exhale with standing and allow arms to rest to the sides. Repeat twice. Relax into a Rag Doll to counterpose the flat back.

Parsvottanasana: Flank Stretch

Try to keep both legs straight throughout.

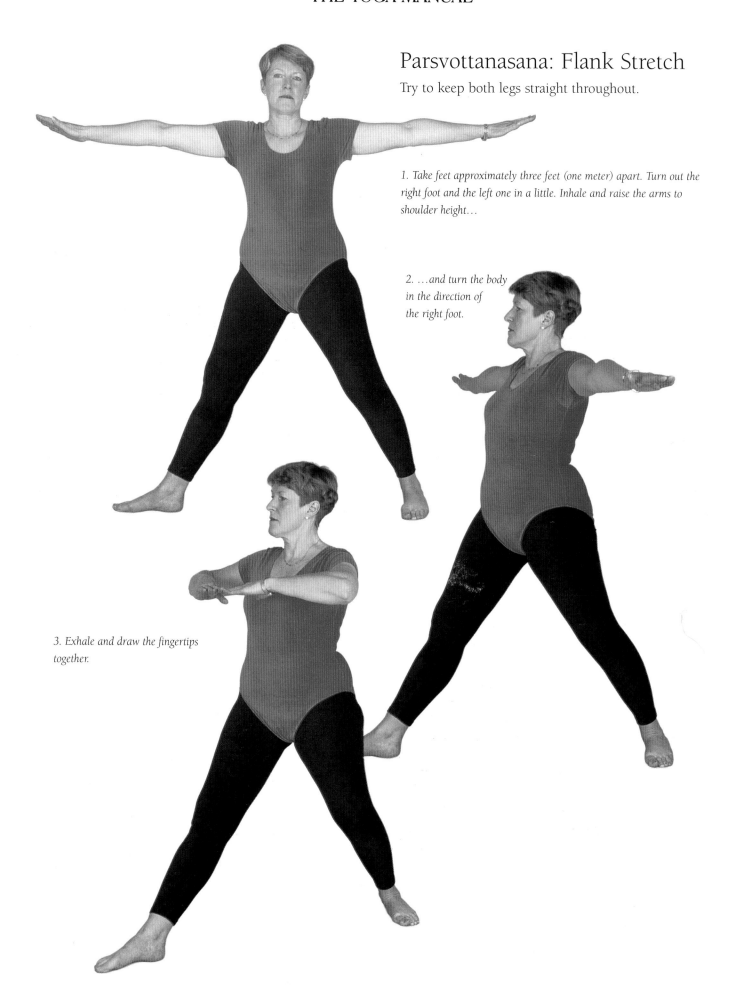

1. *Take feet approximately three feet (one meter) apart. Turn out the right foot and the left one in a little. Inhale and raise the arms to shoulder height…*

2. *…and turn the body in the direction of the right foot.*

3. *Exhale and draw the fingertips together.*

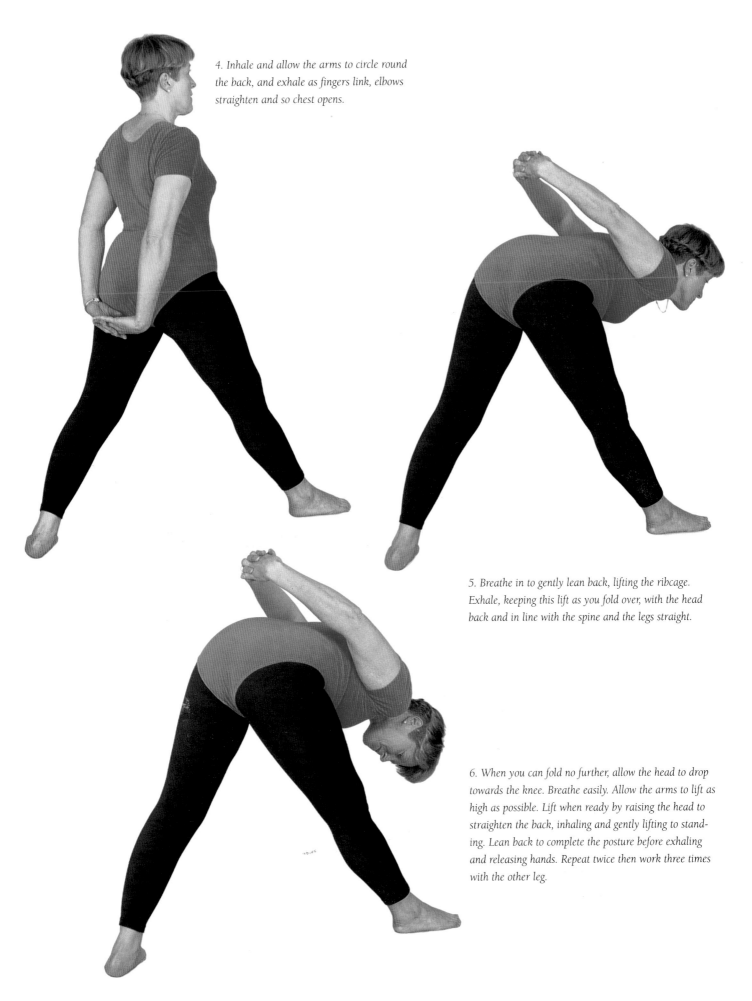

4. Inhale and allow the arms to circle round the back, and exhale as fingers link, elbows straighten and so chest opens.

5. Breathe in to gently lean back, lifting the ribcage. Exhale, keeping this lift as you fold over, with the head back and in line with the spine and the legs straight.

6. When you can fold no further, allow the head to drop towards the knee. Breathe easily. Allow the arms to lift as high as possible. Lift when ready by raising the head to straighten the back, inhaling and gently lifting to standing. Lean back to complete the posture before exhaling and releasing hands. Repeat twice then work three times with the other leg.

Virabhadrasana I: Hero Posture

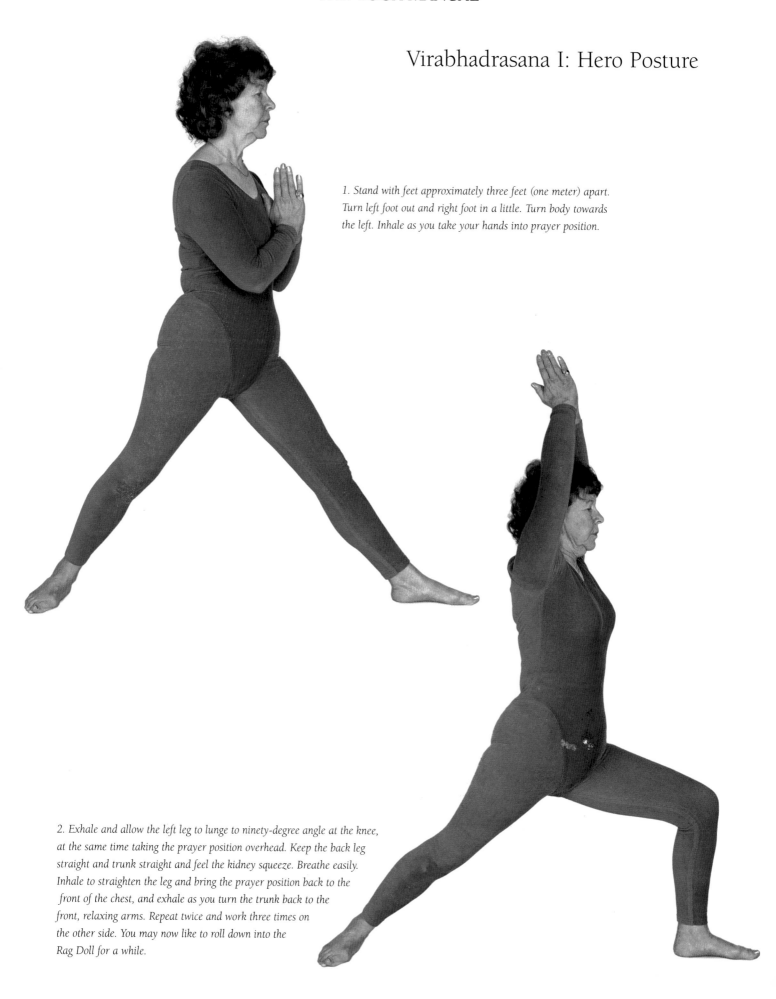

1. Stand with feet approximately three feet (one meter) apart. Turn left foot out and right foot in a little. Turn body towards the left. Inhale as you take your hands into prayer position.

2. Exhale and allow the left leg to lunge to ninety-degree angle at the knee, at the same time taking the prayer position overhead. Keep the back leg straight and trunk straight and feel the kidney squeeze. Breathe easily. Inhale to straighten the leg and bring the prayer position back to the front of the chest, and exhale as you turn the trunk back to the front, relaxing arms. Repeat twice and work three times on the other side. You may now like to roll down into the Rag Doll for a while.

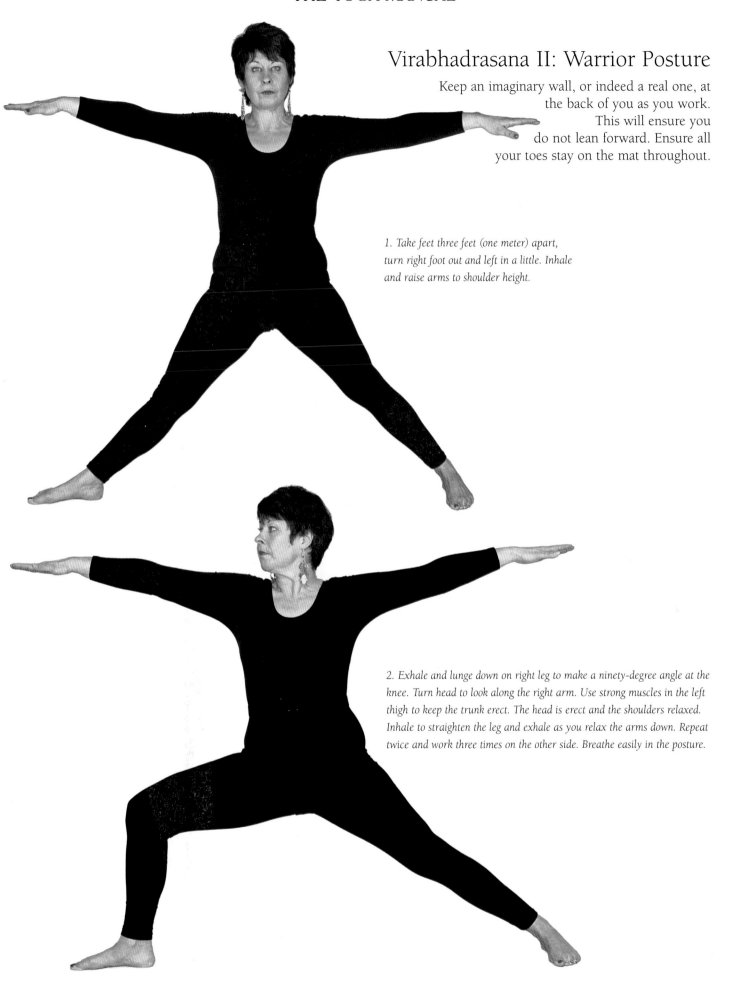

Virabhadrasana II: Warrior Posture

Keep an imaginary wall, or indeed a real one, at
the back of you as you work.
This will ensure you
do not lean forward. Ensure all
your toes stay on the mat throughout.

*1. Take feet three feet (one meter) apart,
turn right foot out and left in a little. Inhale
and raise arms to shoulder height.*

*2. Exhale and lunge down on right leg to make a ninety-degree angle at the
knee. Turn head to look along the right arm. Use strong muscles in the left
thigh to keep the trunk erect. The head is erect and the shoulders relaxed.
Inhale to straighten the leg and exhale as you relax the arms down. Repeat
twice and work three times on the other side. Breathe easily in the posture.*

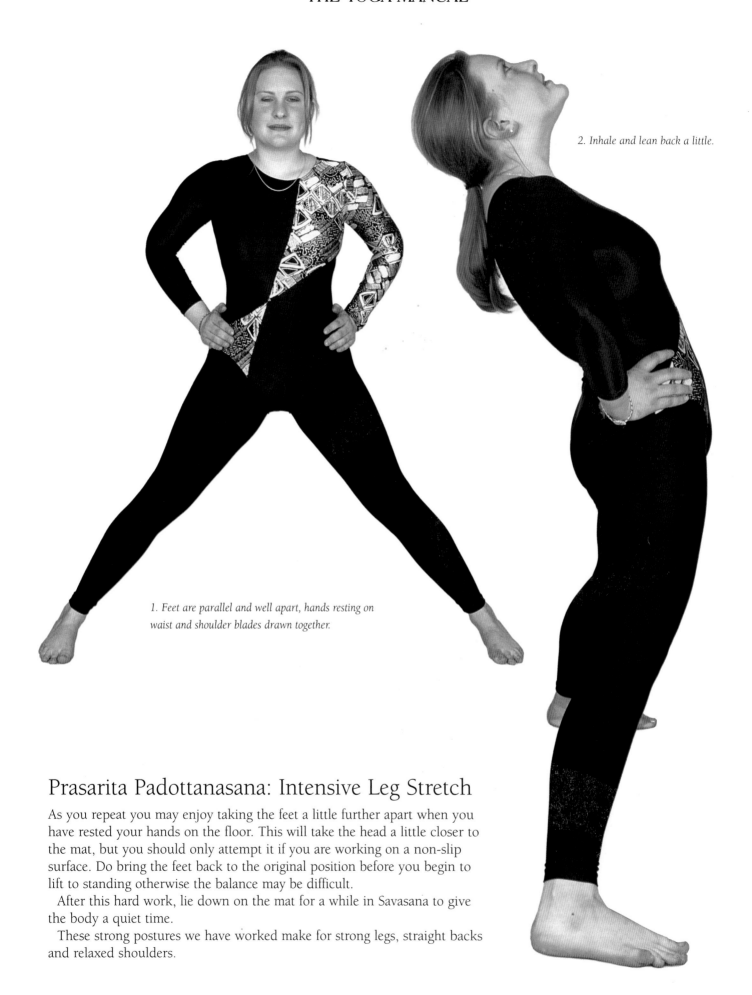

2. Inhale and lean back a little.

1. Feet are parallel and well apart, hands resting on waist and shoulder blades drawn together.

Prasarita Padottanasana: Intensive Leg Stretch

As you repeat you may enjoy taking the feet a little further apart when you have rested your hands on the floor. This will take the head a little closer to the mat, but you should only attempt it if you are working on a non-slip surface. Do bring the feet back to the original position before you begin to lift to standing otherwise the balance may be difficult.

After this hard work, lie down on the mat for a while in Savasana to give the body a quiet time.

These strong postures we have worked make for strong legs, straight backs and relaxed shoulders.

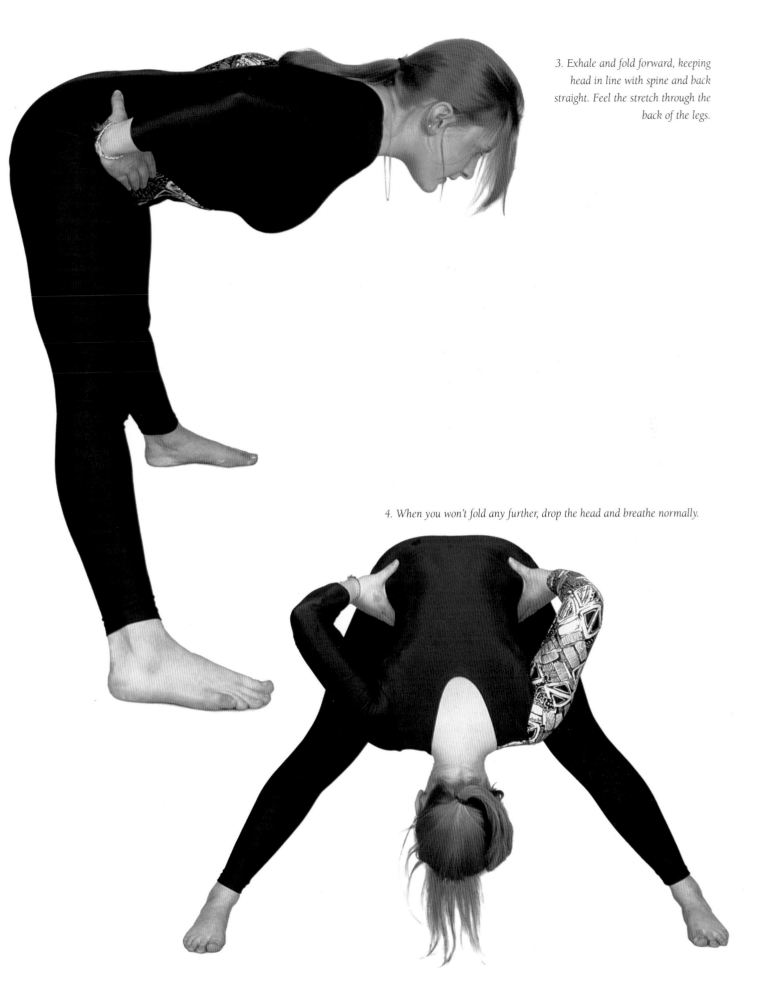

3. Exhale and fold forward, keeping head in line with spine and back straight. Feel the stretch through the back of the legs.

4. When you won't fold any further, drop the head and breathe normally.

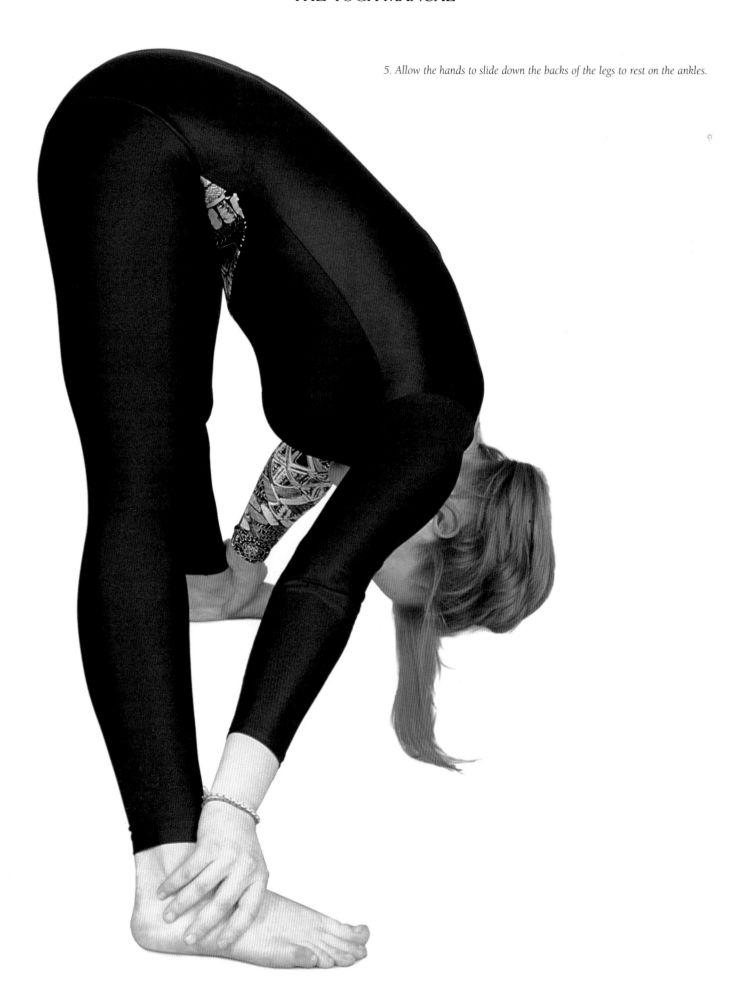

5. Allow the hands to slide down the backs of the legs to rest on the ankles.

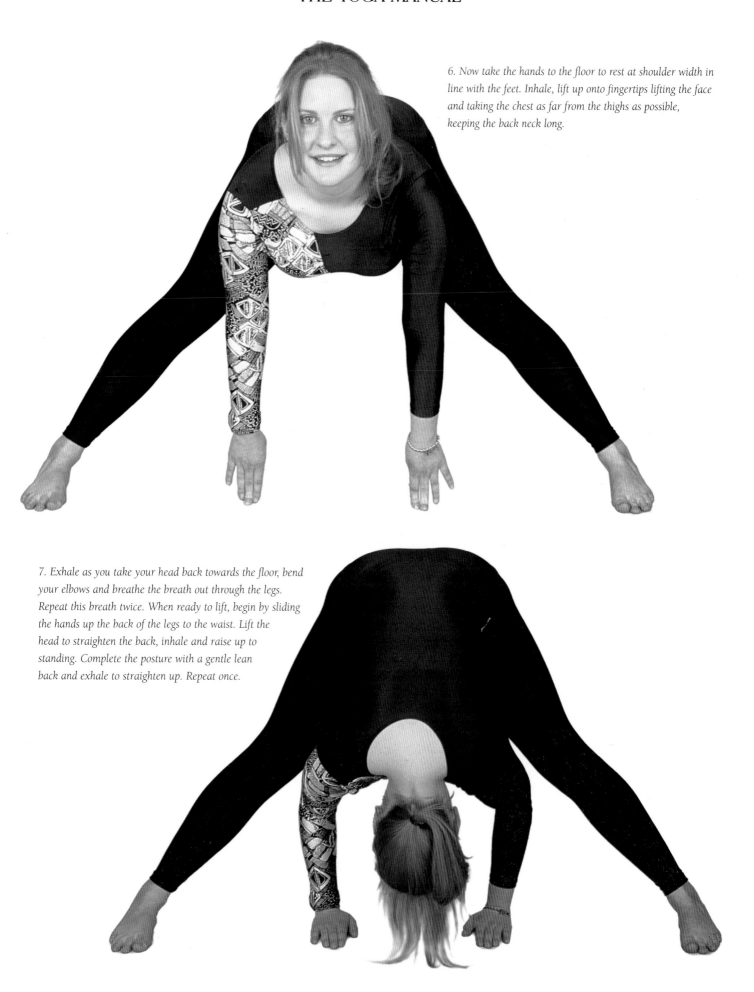

6. Now take the hands to the floor to rest at shoulder width in line with the feet. Inhale, lift up onto fingertips lifting the face and taking the chest as far from the thighs as possible, keeping the back neck long.

7. Exhale as you take your head back towards the floor, bend your elbows and breathe the breath out through the legs. Repeat this breath twice. When ready to lift, begin by sliding the hands up the back of the legs to the waist. Lift the head to straighten the back, inhale and raise up to standing. Complete the posture with a gentle lean back and exhale to straighten up. Repeat once.

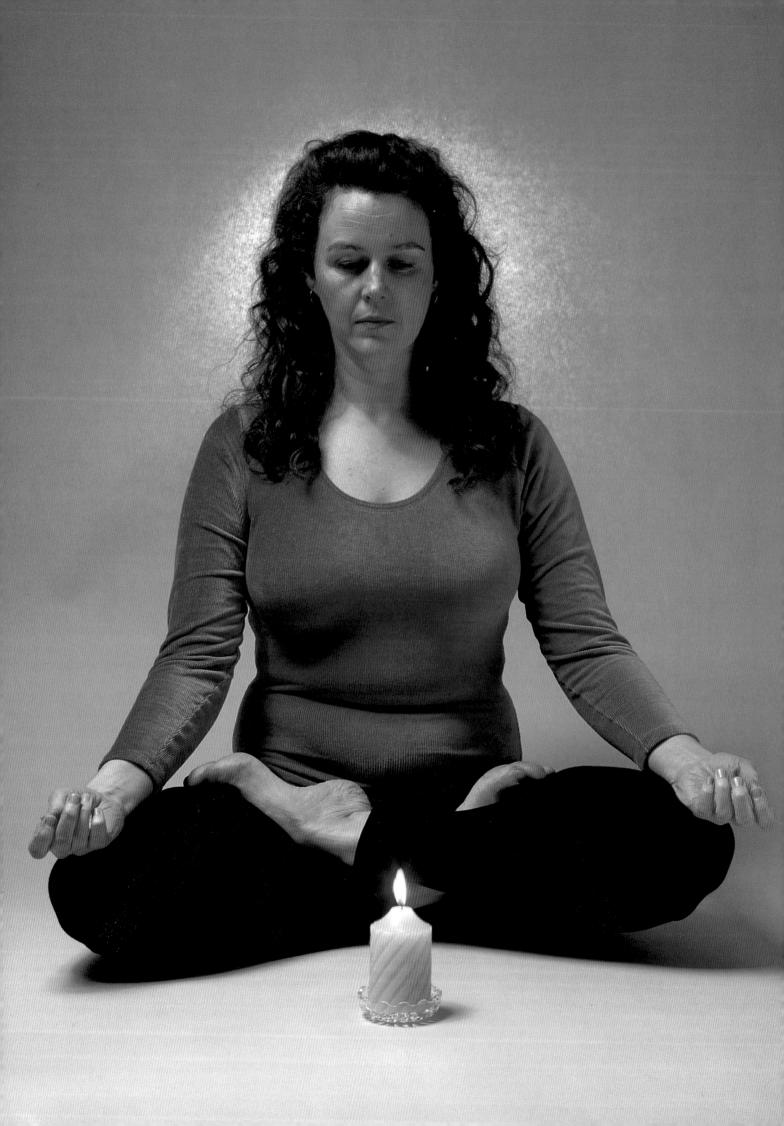

Parivrtta Trikonasana: Twisted Triangle

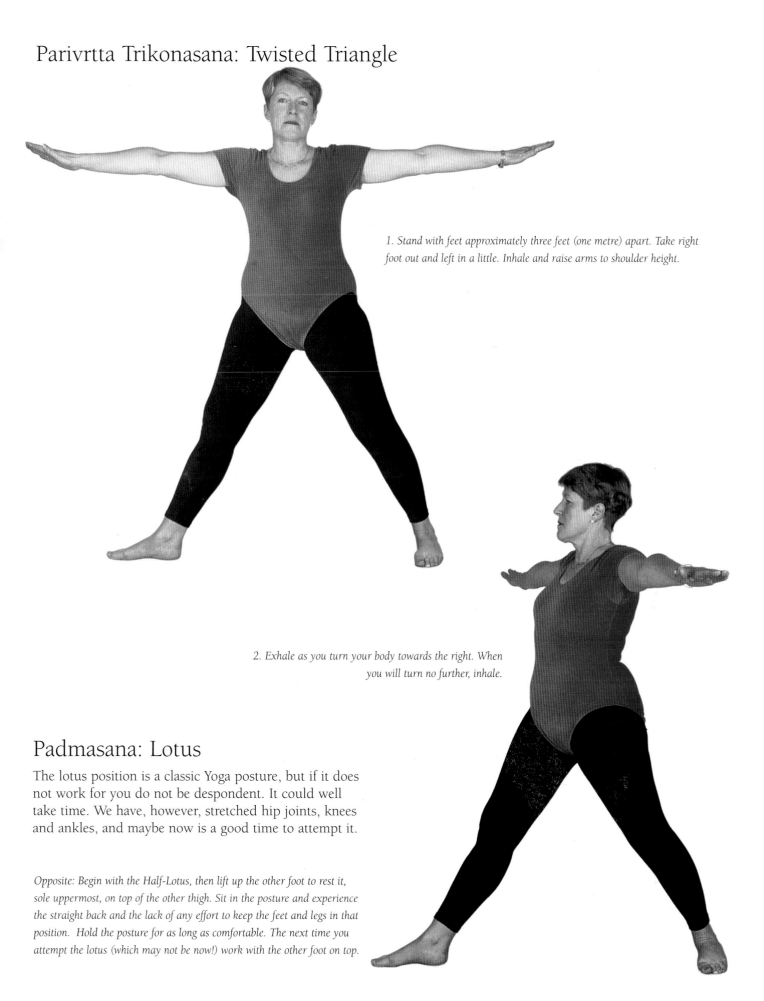

1. Stand with feet approximately three feet (one metre) apart. Take right foot out and left in a little. Inhale and raise arms to shoulder height.

2. Exhale as you turn your body towards the right. When you will turn no further, inhale.

Padmasana: Lotus

The lotus position is a classic Yoga posture, but if it does not work for you do not be despondent. It could well take time. We have, however, stretched hip joints, knees and ankles, and maybe now is a good time to attempt it.

Opposite: Begin with the Half-Lotus, then lift up the other foot to rest it, sole uppermost, on top of the other thigh. Sit in the posture and experience the straight back and the lack of any effort to keep the feet and legs in that position. Hold the posture for as long as comfortable. The next time you attempt the lotus (which may not be now!) work with the other foot on top.

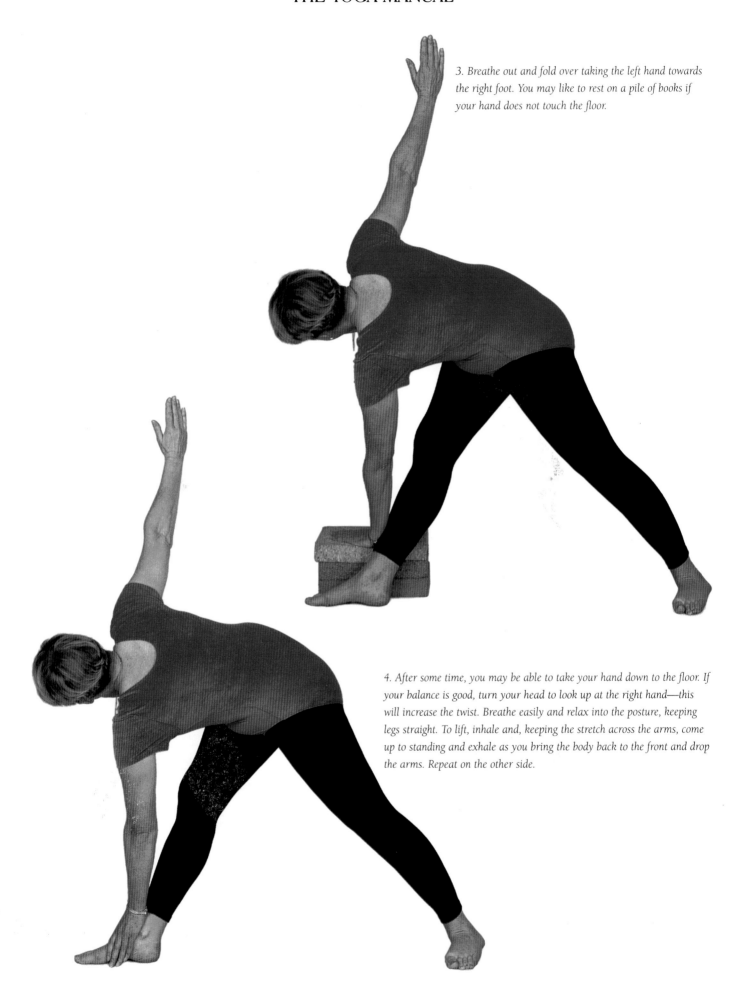

3. Breathe out and fold over taking the left hand towards the right foot. You may like to rest on a pile of books if your hand does not touch the floor.

4. After some time, you may be able to take your hand down to the floor. If your balance is good, turn your head to look up at the right hand—this will increase the twist. Breathe easily and relax into the posture, keeping legs straight. To lift, inhale and, keeping the stretch across the arms, come up to standing and exhale as you bring the body back to the front and drop the arms. Repeat on the other side.

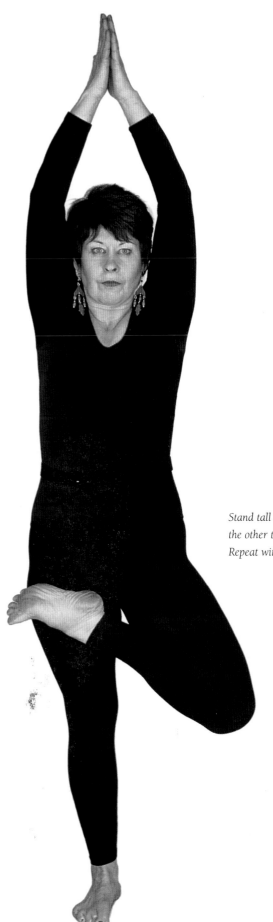

Vrksasana: Half-Lotus Tree Balance

Feel you lift to the sky as you balance, but feel the shoulders relax.

Yoga Nidra: Total Relaxation

This Yoga has been hard work so you really deserve a long relaxation. Yield to your mat, take your awareness through the whole of the body to relax and soothe it. Listen to the soft music as you sink down into the floor. I am at ease. I am at peace. I am relaxed.

Visualize yourself now lying on a beach by the waters edge. You are warm and relaxed. Your eyes are closed but you know the sun is bright and the sky is blue. As you inhale a gentle wave of warm, soft water completely engulfs you. As you exhale, that water ebbs away taking with it any traces of tension or negativity left in your body. Continue with this pleasant visualization for a few minutes …

Begin to let the breath deepen. Stretch and yawn when you feel ready, roll over to the right side and sit up. Before opening your eyes, run your fingertips lightly over your closed eyelids.

Stand tall and fix your gaze. Lift a foot to rest, sole uppermost, at the top of the other thigh. Take the hands into prayer position and stretch overhead. Repeat with the other leg.

Yoga is an open—ing of silence
Within the mind;
The dissolution of clouds
In the pool of clarity
And allowing passage
To the winds of space.
Yoga is the arising of smile
From the roots of silence;
The play of sunlight
On the open petals
And allowing passage
To the breath of grace.

—Velta Snikere Wilson

CHAPTER SEVEN

LIVING WITH YOGA

This chapter provides a series of simple sessions in an easy-to-follow format that will help you to integrate Yoga into your life. By doing one or more of these sessions each day, you will be able to increase your flexibility and ease the effects of stress on your body and your mind.

Surya Namaskar: Salute to the Sun

Sometimes you may not have time to do a whole Yoga session, but you may have time for just one round of salute to the sun. When you know the sequence well you will be able to allow it to flow quite quickly and find it very vitalizing.

Stage 1. Begin by standing tall with hands in prayer position.

Stage 2. Inhale and stretch arms overhead and lean back, looking to the sun.

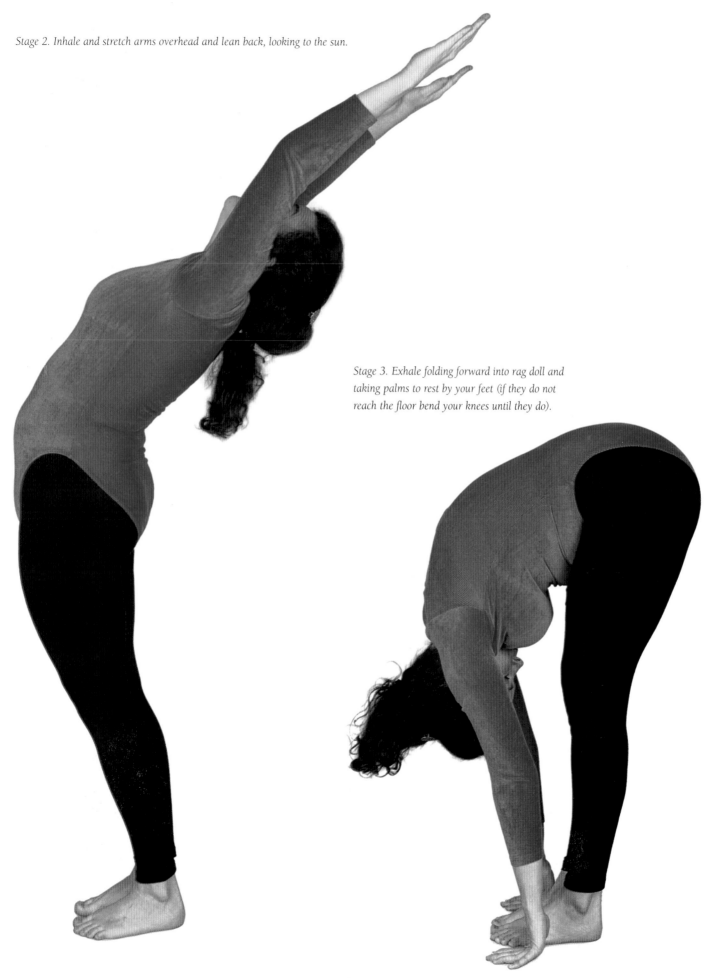

Stage 3. Exhale folding forward into rag doll and taking palms to rest by your feet (if they do not reach the floor bend your knees until they do).

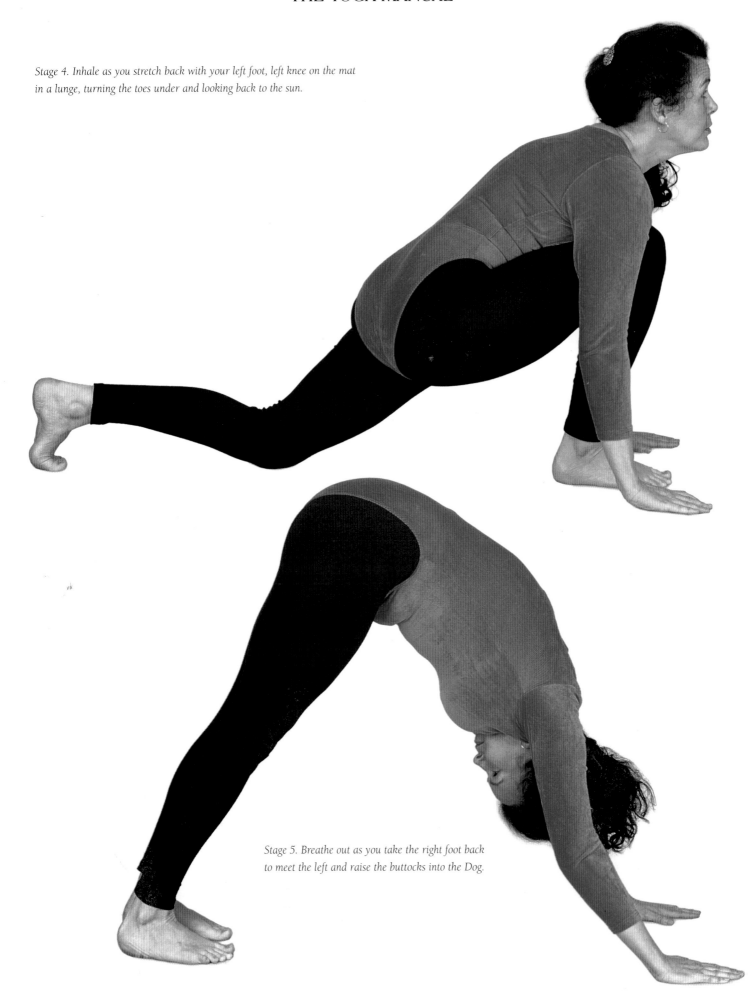

Stage 4. Inhale as you stretch back with your left foot, left knee on the mat in a lunge, turning the toes under and looking back to the sun.

Stage 5. Breathe out as you take the right foot back to meet the left and raise the buttocks into the Dog.

Stage 6. Hold the breath out as you bring the knees, chest and chin onto the mat, leaving the bottom pushed up.

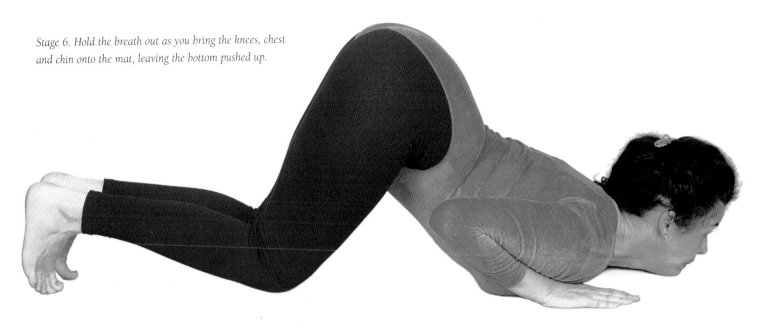

Stage 7. Inhale and slide the body forward through the hands into a raised Cobra, resting just on the hands and toes. Look back to the sun.

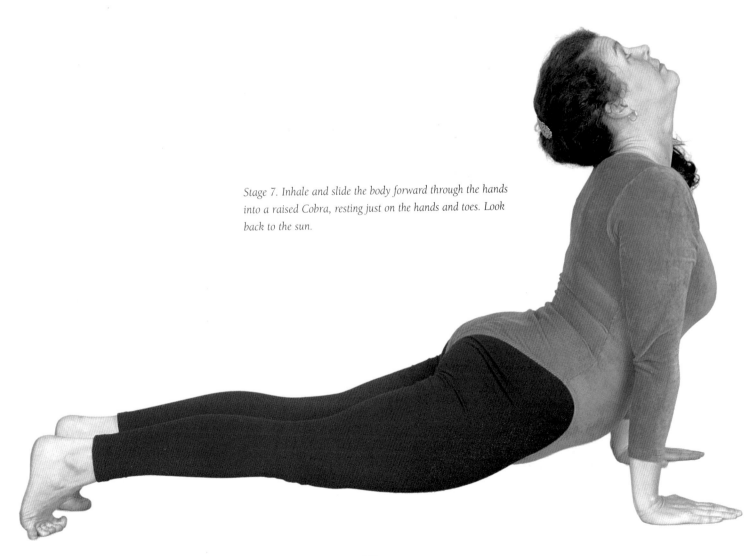

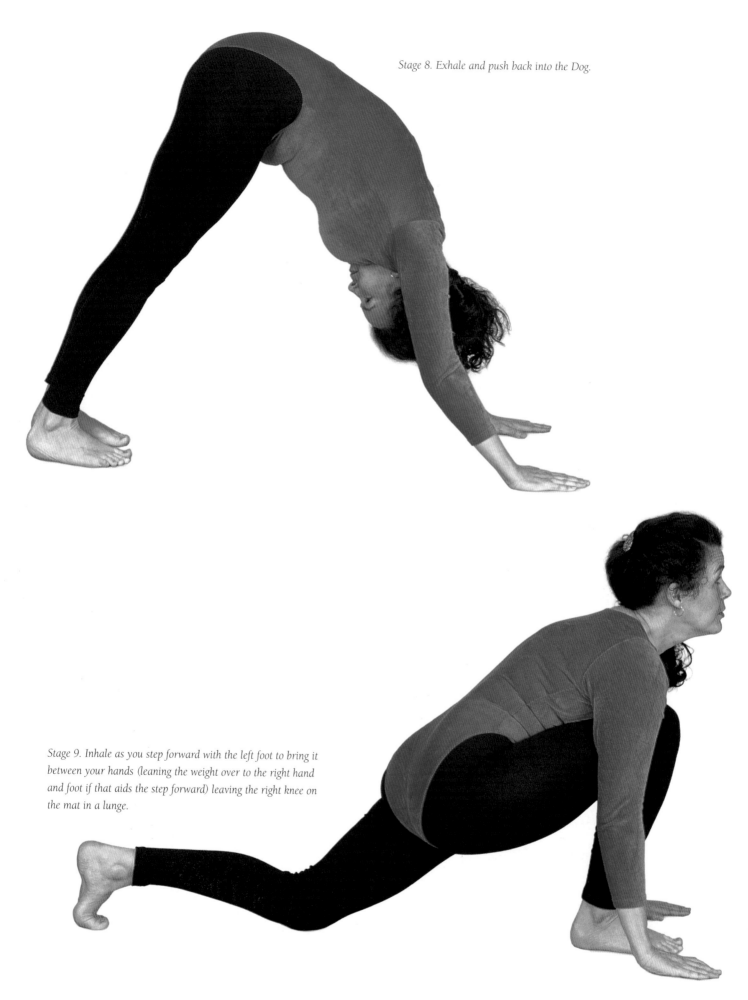

Stage 8. Exhale and push back into the Dog.

Stage 9. Inhale as you step forward with the left foot to bring it between your hands (leaning the weight over to the right hand and foot if that aids the step forward) leaving the right knee on the mat in a lunge.

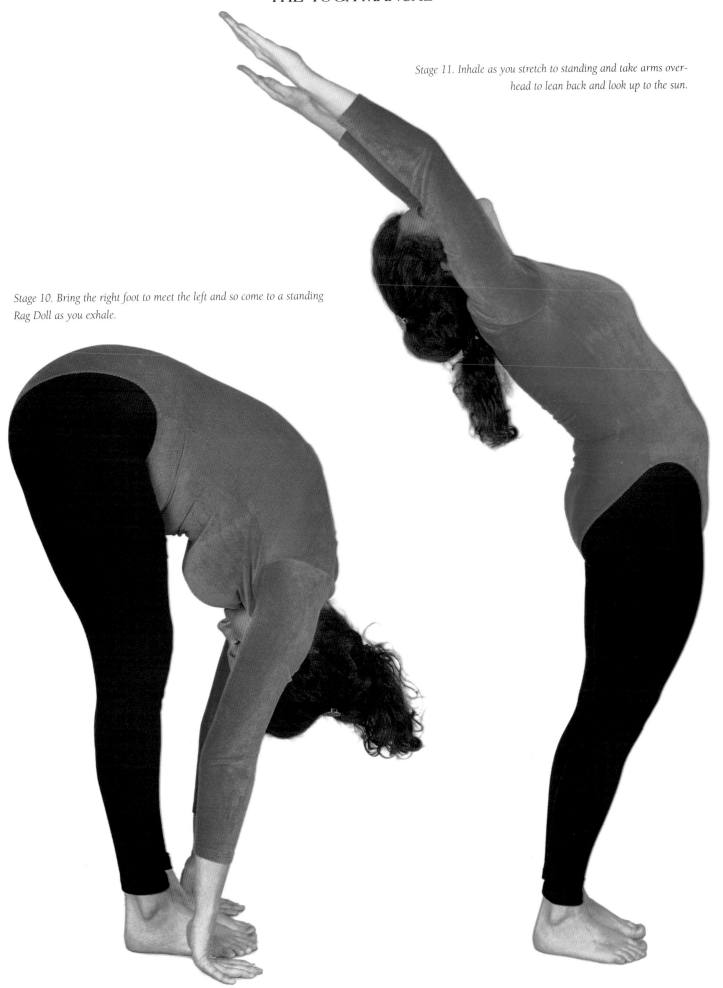

Stage 11. Inhale as you stretch to standing and take arms overhead to lean back and look up to the sun.

Stage 10. Bring the right foot to meet the left and so come to a standing Rag Doll as you exhale.

Stage 12. You have now completed a round of Salute to the Sun. Repeat but by taking the right leg back in Stage 4 and bringing the right foot forward in Stage 9. Exhale as you bring the hands back to Prayer Position.

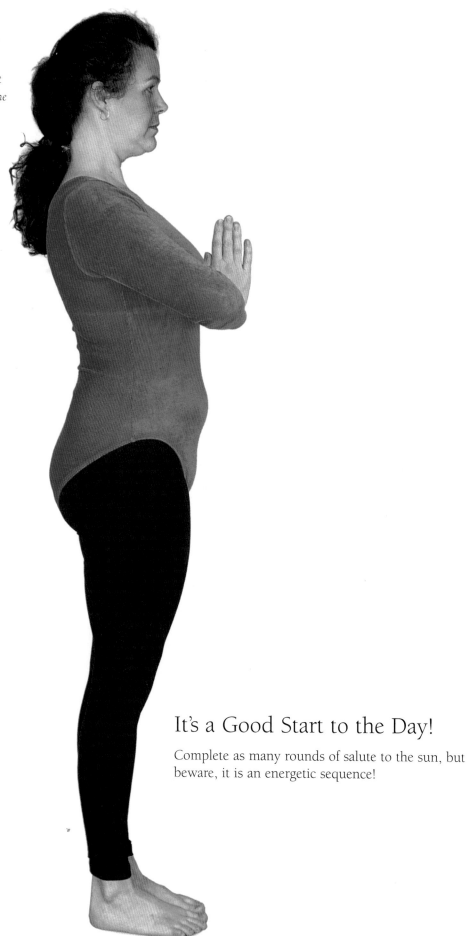

It's a Good Start to the Day!

Complete as many rounds of salute to the sun, but beware, it is an energetic sequence!

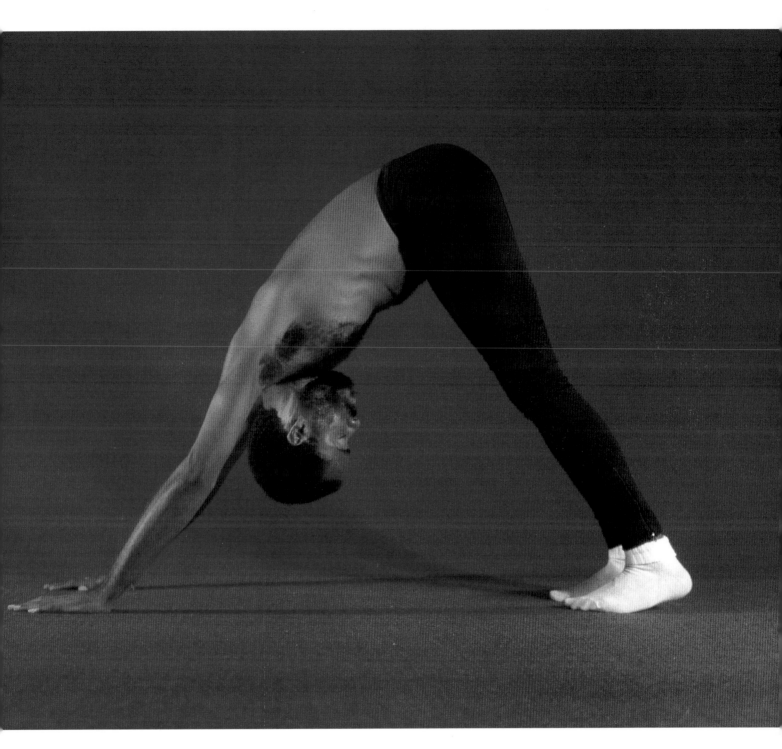

Above: Part of the Sun Sequence

Forward Bend/Plough Sequence

This sequence seems to work best if it is kept perpetually moving with the breath.

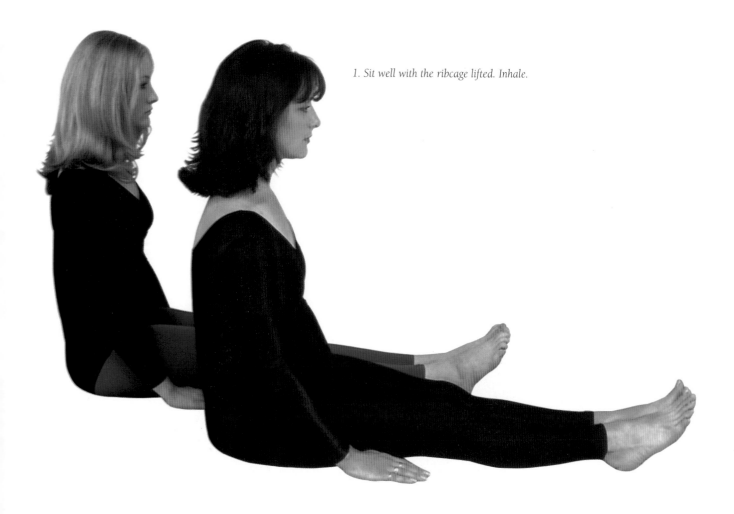

1. Sit well with the ribcage lifted. Inhale.

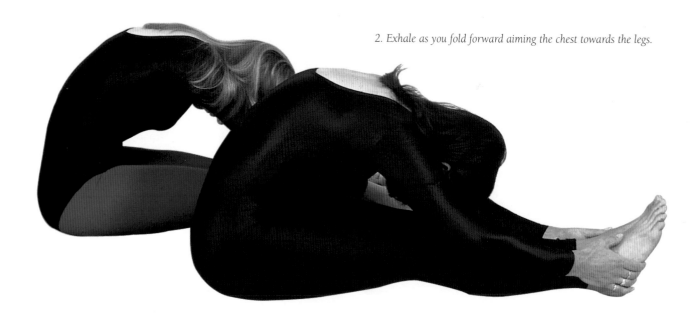

2. Exhale as you fold forward aiming the chest towards the legs.

3. Inhale to sit up again.

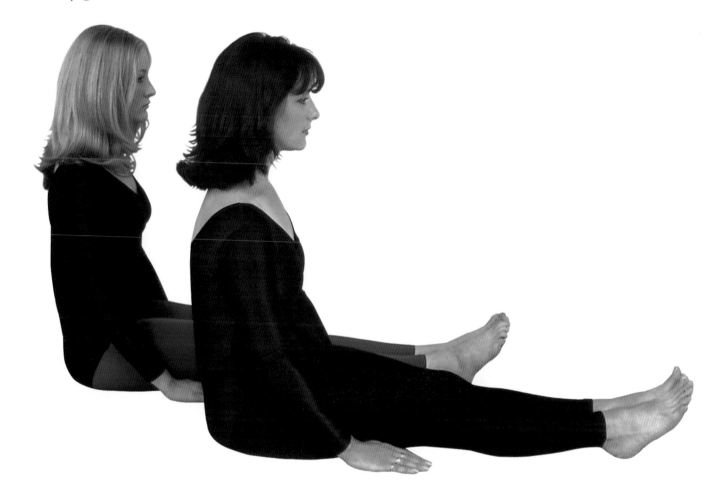

4. Exhale to roll the spine down to the floor.

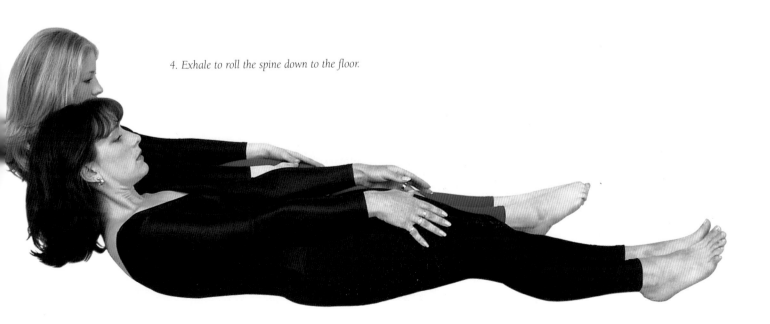

5. *Inhale to bend the knees and raise the feet towards the ceiling.*

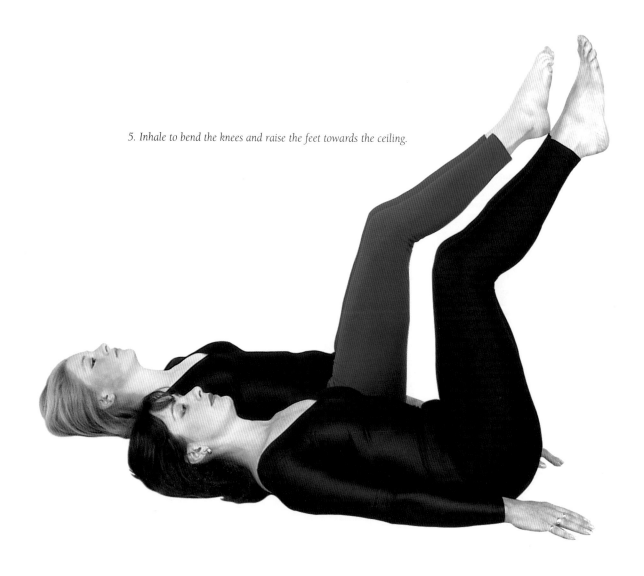

6. *Exhale to fold over into the Plough (maybe using a chair or blocks to rest the feet).*

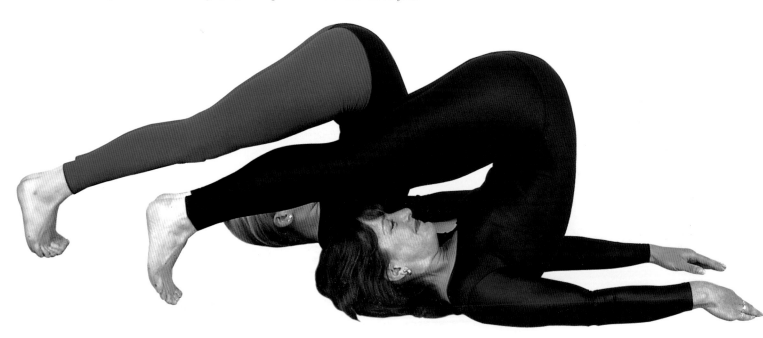

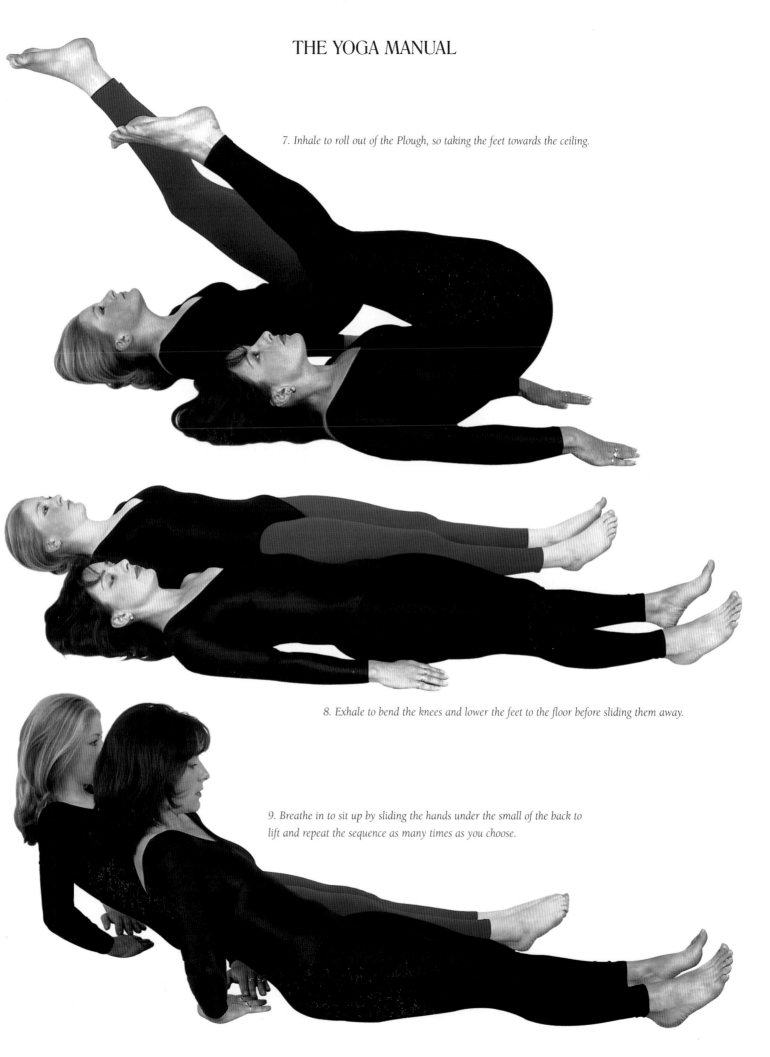

7. *Inhale to roll out of the Plough, so taking the feet towards the ceiling.*

8. *Exhale to bend the knees and lower the feet to the floor before sliding them away.*

9. *Breathe in to sit up by sliding the hands under the small of the back to lift and repeat the sequence as many times as you choose.*

Yoga at a Glance

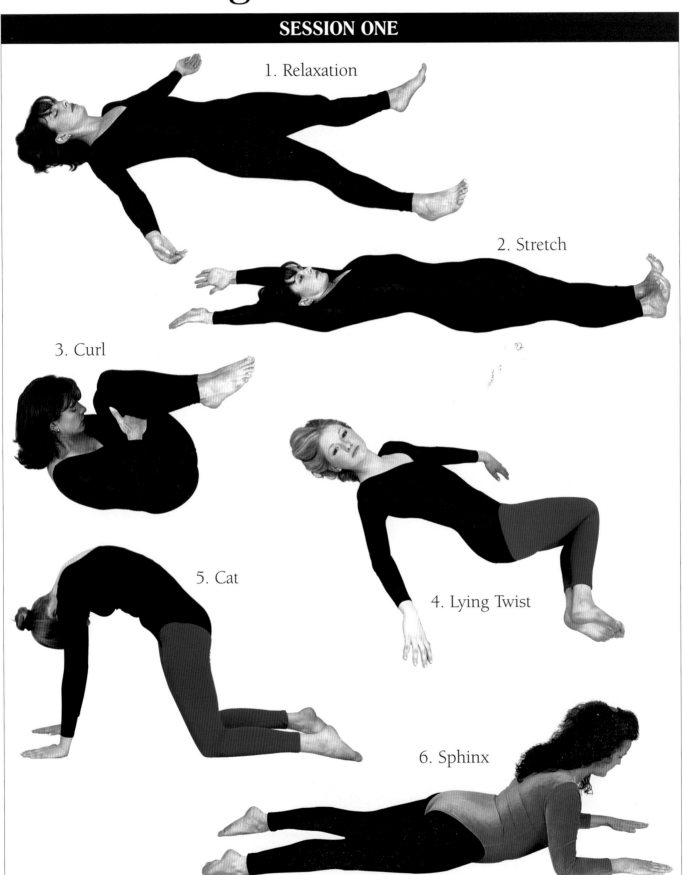

1. Relaxation

2. Stretch

3. Curl

5. Cat

4. Lying Twist

6. Sphinx

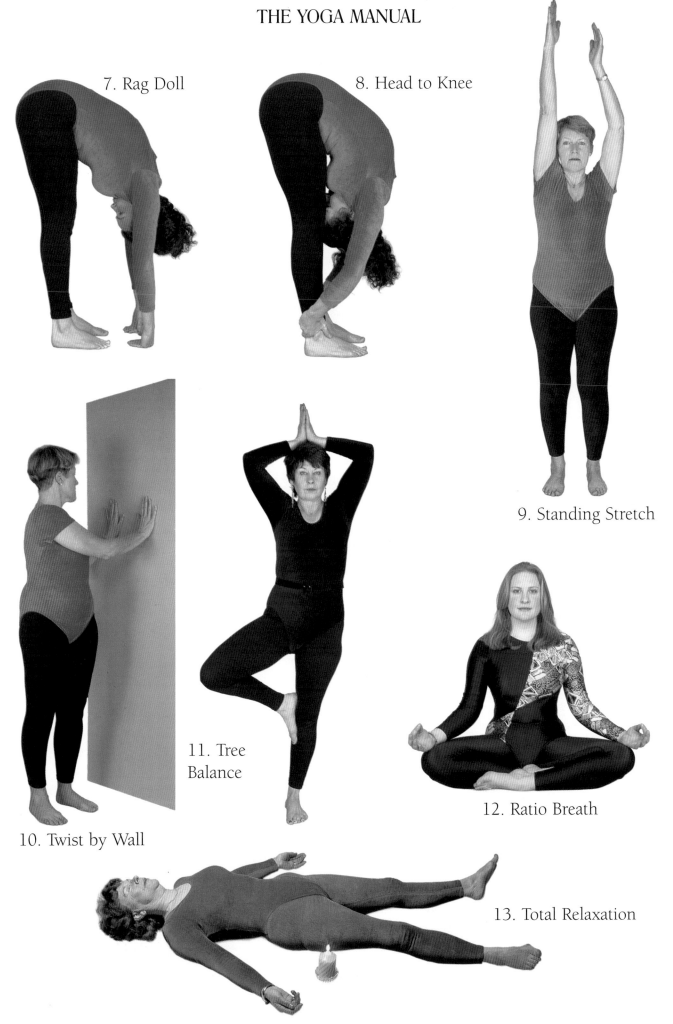

7. Rag Doll

8. Head to Knee

9. Standing Stretch

11. Tree Balance

10. Twist by Wall

12. Ratio Breath

13. Total Relaxation

SESSION TWO

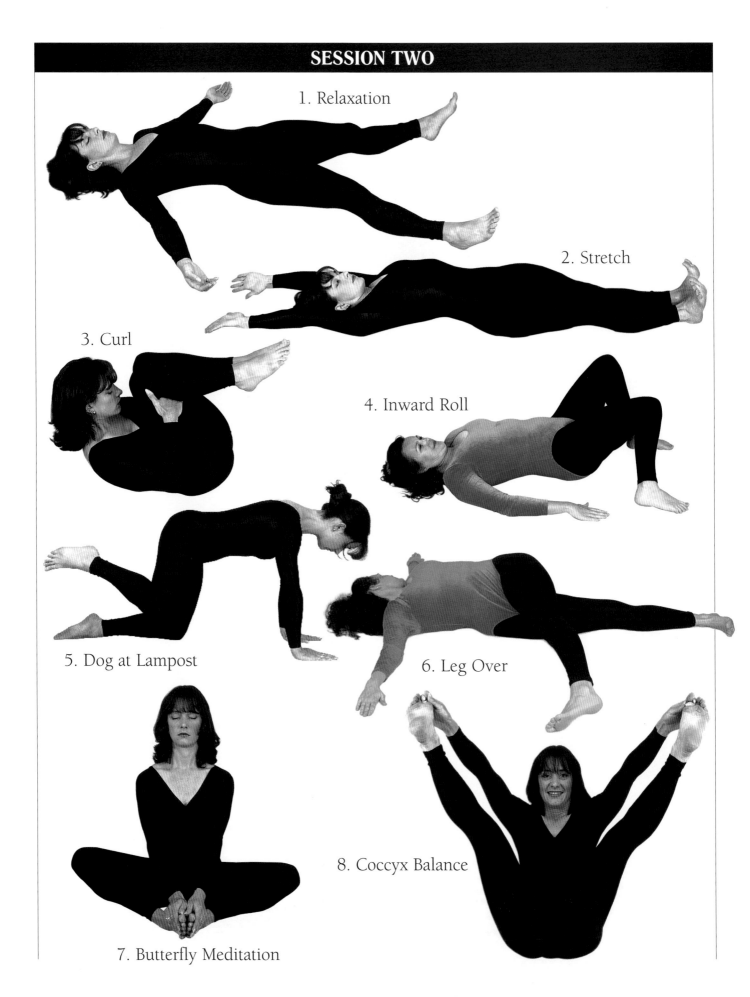

1. Relaxation

2. Stretch

3. Curl

4. Inward Roll

5. Dog at Lampost

6. Leg Over

7. Butterfly Meditation

8. Coccyx Balance

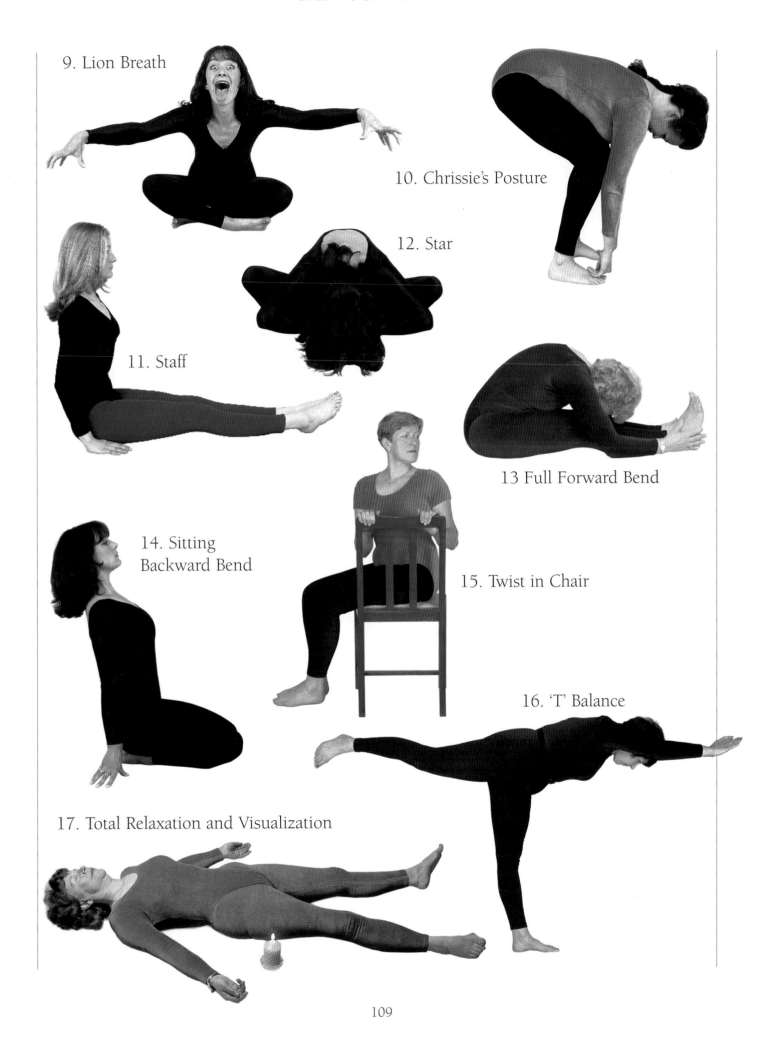

9. Lion Breath

10. Chrissie's Posture

12. Star

11. Staff

13 Full Forward Bend

14. Sitting Backward Bend

15. Twist in Chair

16. 'T' Balance

17. Total Relaxation and Visualization

SESSION THREE

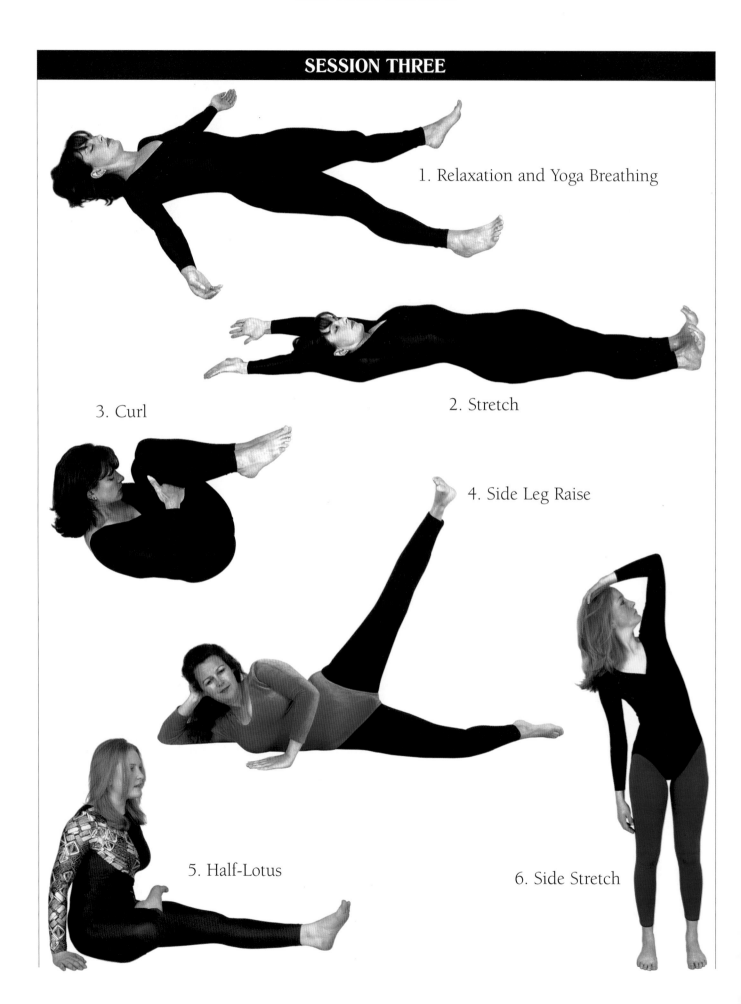

1. Relaxation and Yoga Breathing

2. Stretch

3. Curl

4. Side Leg Raise

5. Half-Lotus

6. Side Stretch

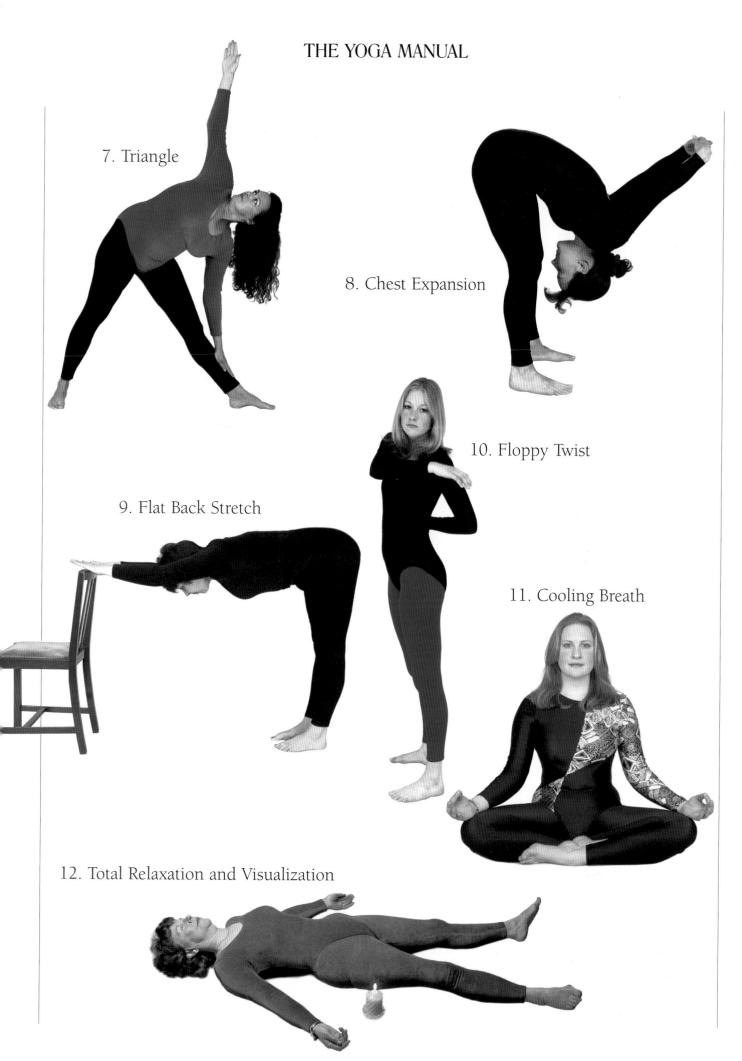

7. Triangle

8. Chest Expansion

9. Flat Back Stretch

10. Floppy Twist

11. Cooling Breath

12. Total Relaxation and Visualization

SESSION FOUR

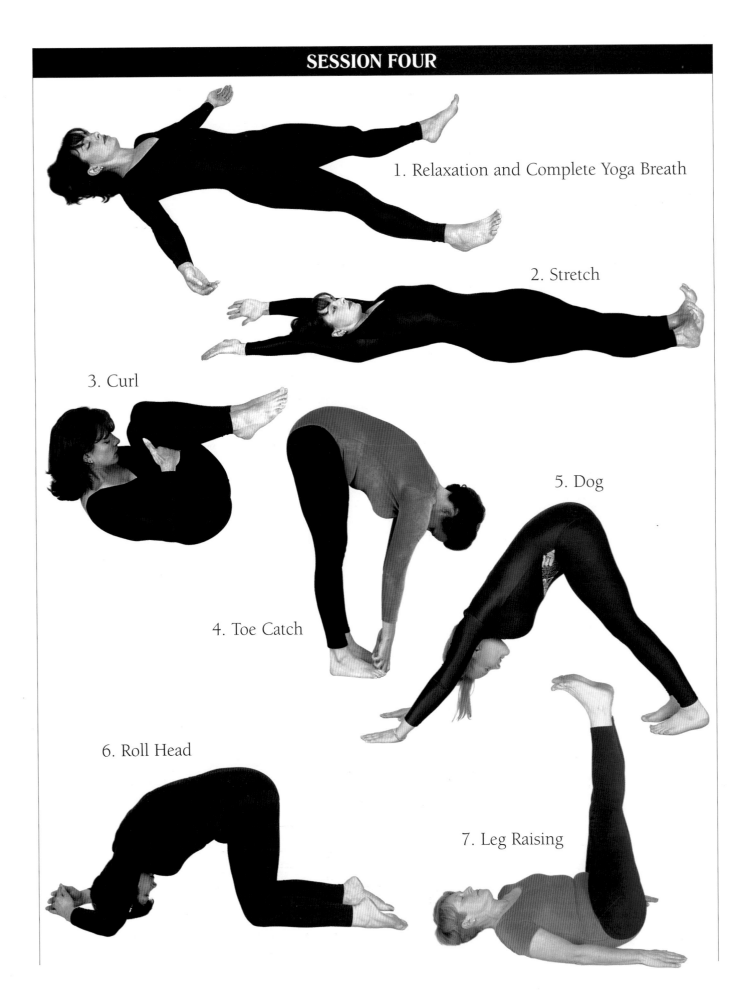

1. Relaxation and Complete Yoga Breath

2. Stretch

3. Curl

4. Toe Catch

5. Dog

6. Roll Head

7. Leg Raising

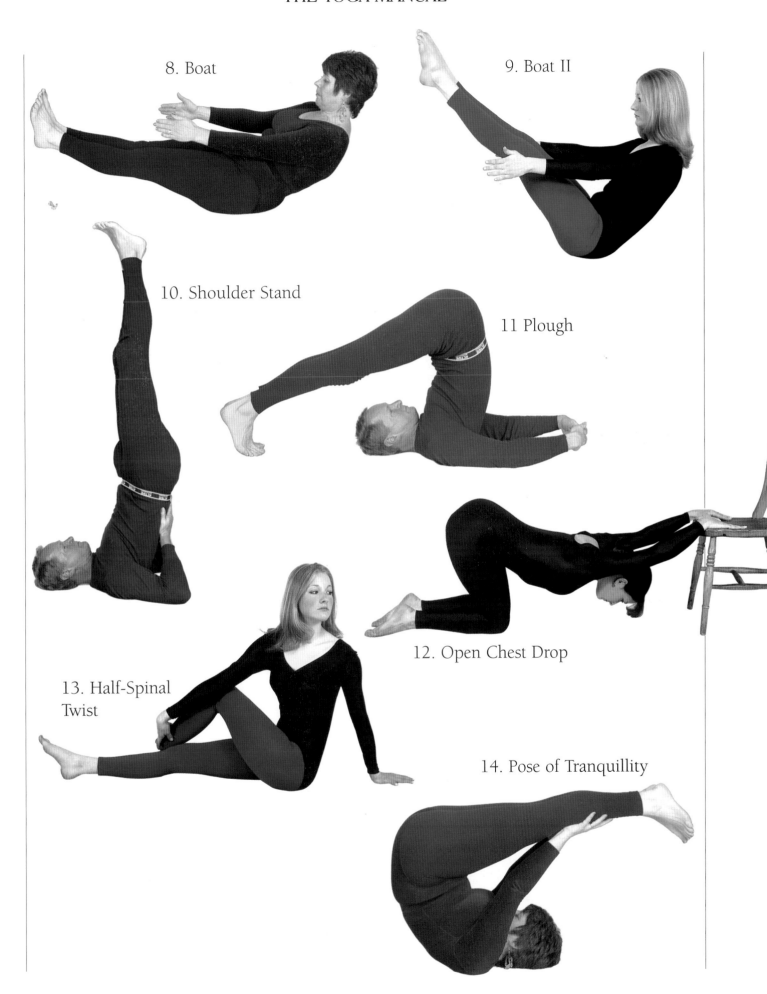

8. Boat

9. Boat II

10. Shoulder Stand

11 Plough

12. Open Chest Drop

13. Half-Spinal Twist

14. Pose of Tranquillity

SESSION FIVE

1. Relaxation and Yoga Breathing

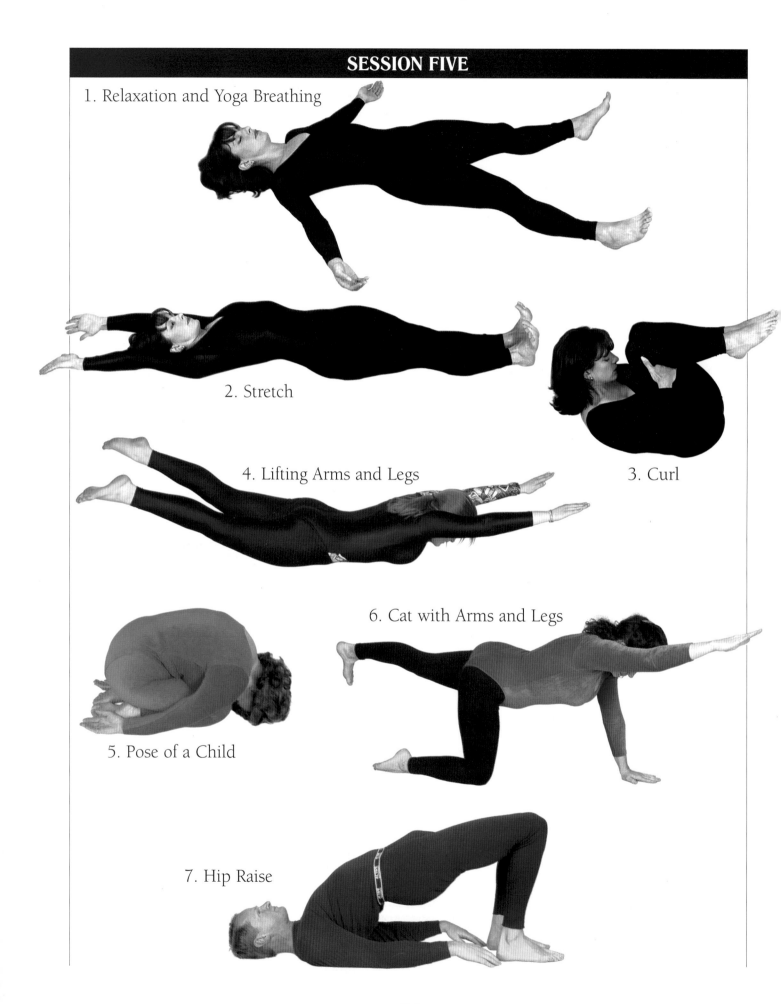

2. Stretch

3. Curl

4. Lifting Arms and Legs

5. Pose of a Child

6. Cat with Arms and Legs

7. Hip Raise

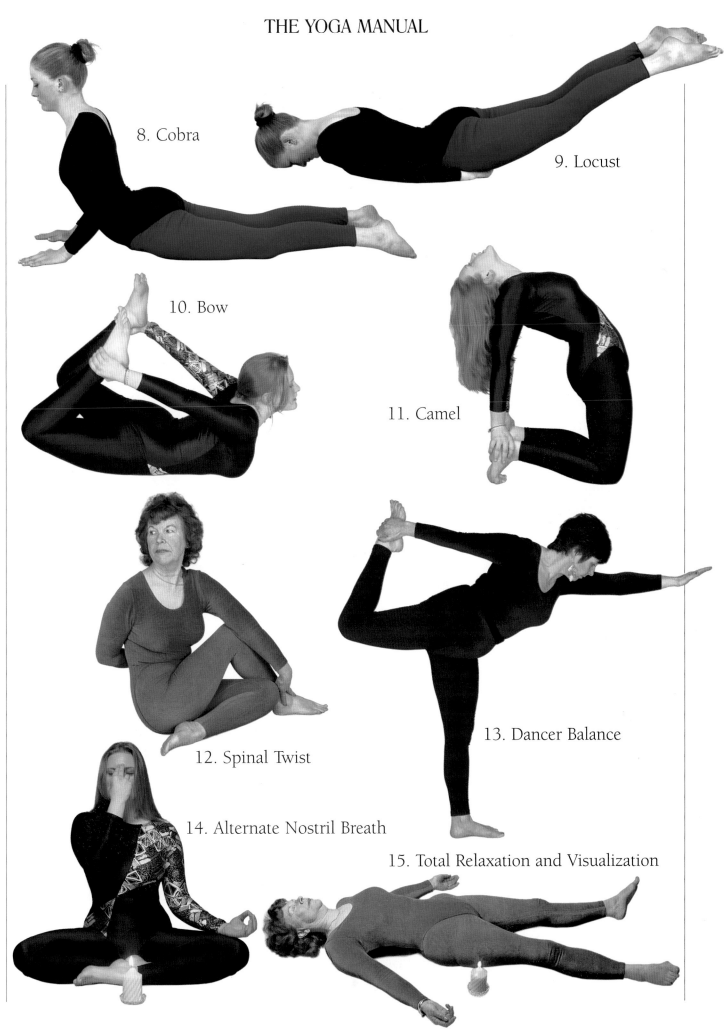

8. Cobra

9. Locust

10. Bow

11. Camel

12. Spinal Twist

13. Dancer Balance

14. Alternate Nostril Breath

15. Total Relaxation and Visualization

SESSION SIX

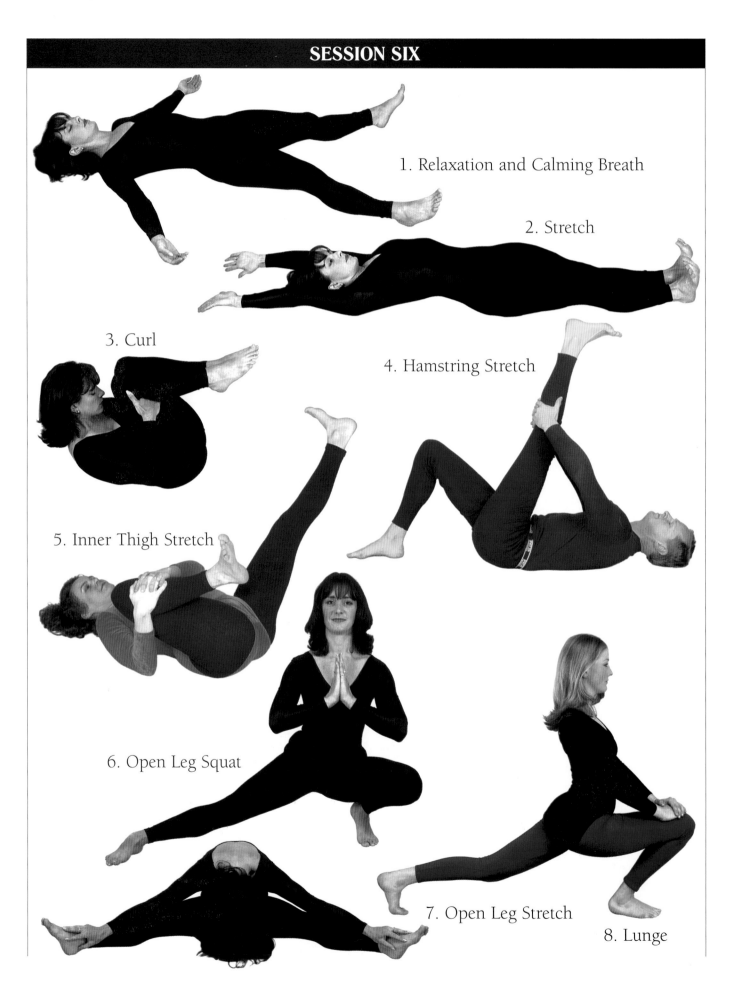

1. Relaxation and Calming Breath

2. Stretch

3. Curl

4. Hamstring Stretch

5. Inner Thigh Stretch

6. Open Leg Squat

7. Open Leg Stretch

8. Lunge

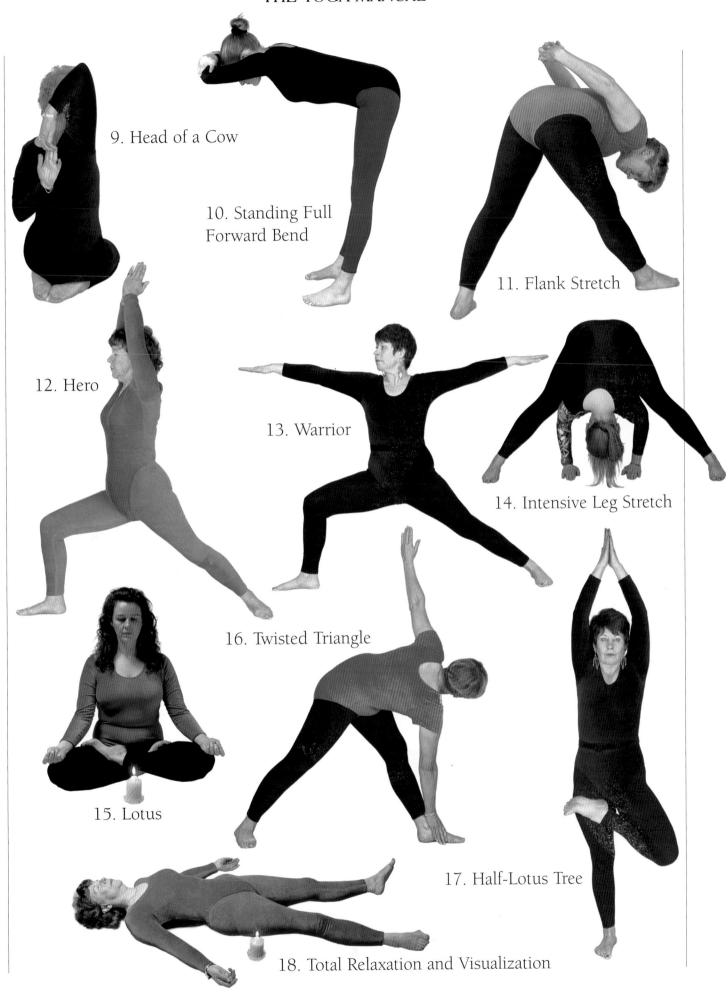

9. Head of a Cow

10. Standing Full
Forward Bend

11. Flank Stretch

12. Hero

13. Warrior

14. Intensive Leg Stretch

16. Twisted Triangle

15. Lotus

17. Half-Lotus Tree

18. Total Relaxation and Visualization

Salute to the Sun

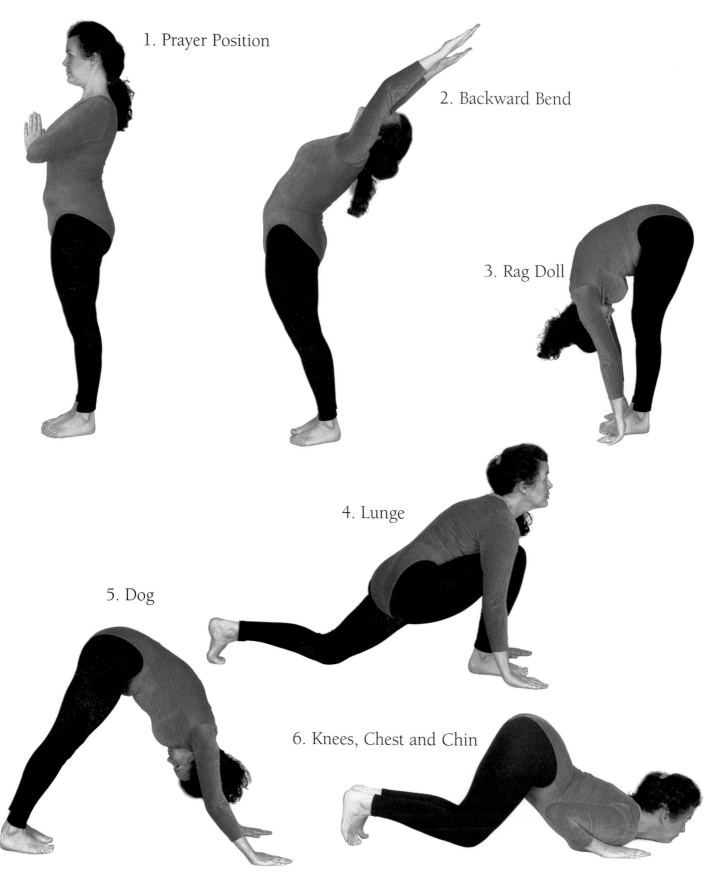

1. Prayer Position

2. Backward Bend

3. Rag Doll

4. Lunge

5. Dog

6. Knees, Chest and Chin

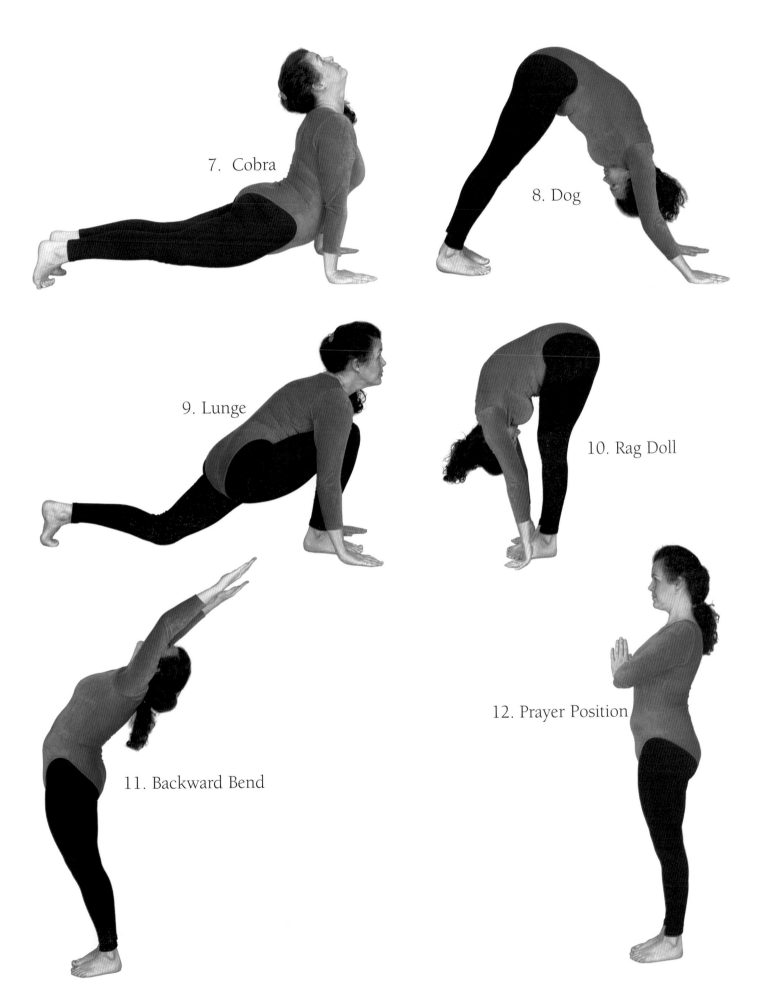

7. Cobra

8. Dog

9. Lunge

10. Rag Doll

11. Backward Bend

12. Prayer Position

Forward Bend/Plough Sequence at a glance

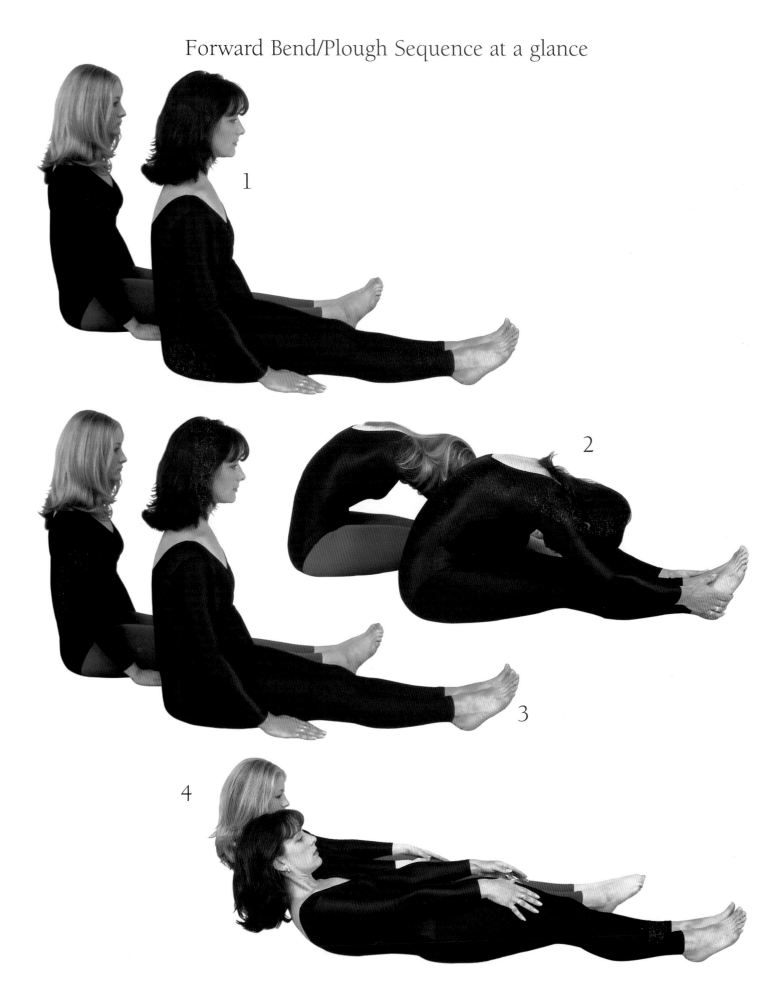

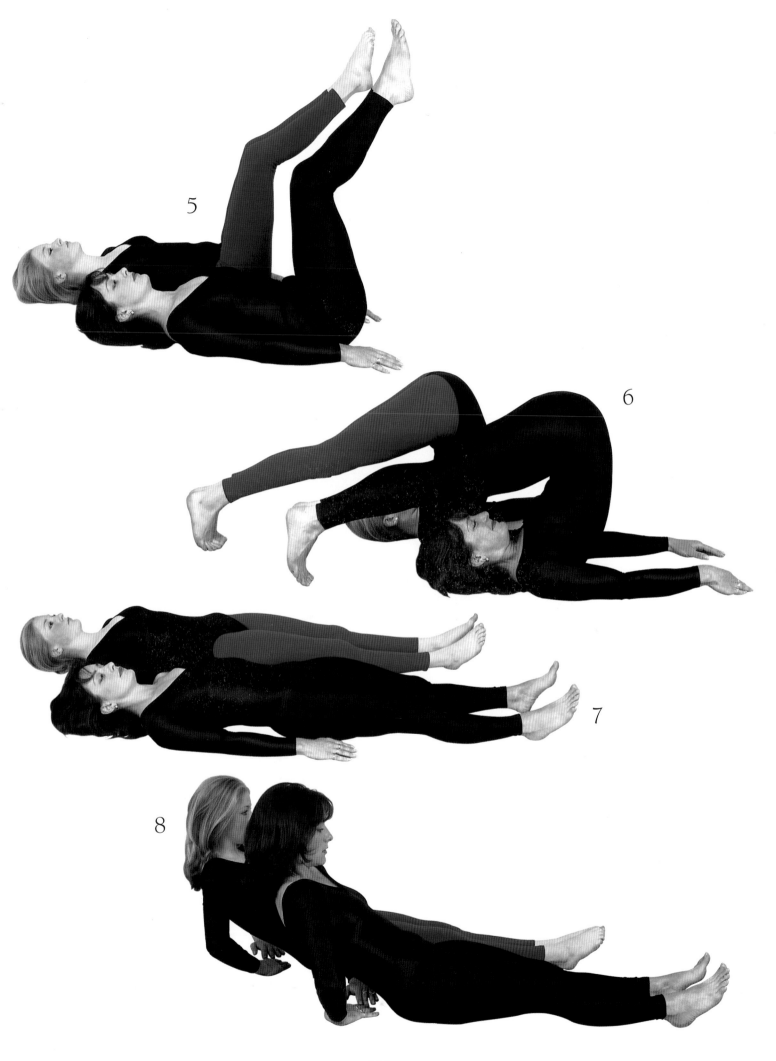

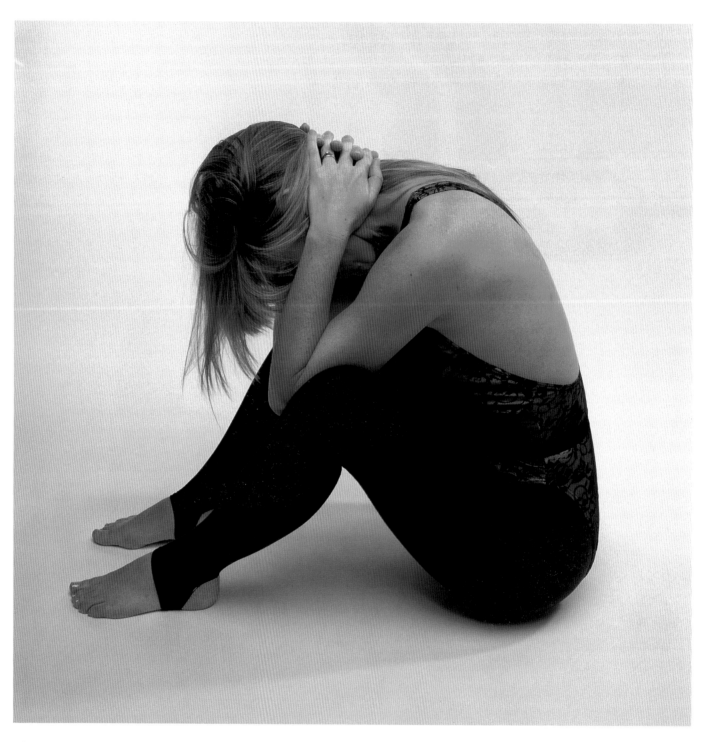

Above: Rounding the back

Opposite: Back neck stretch

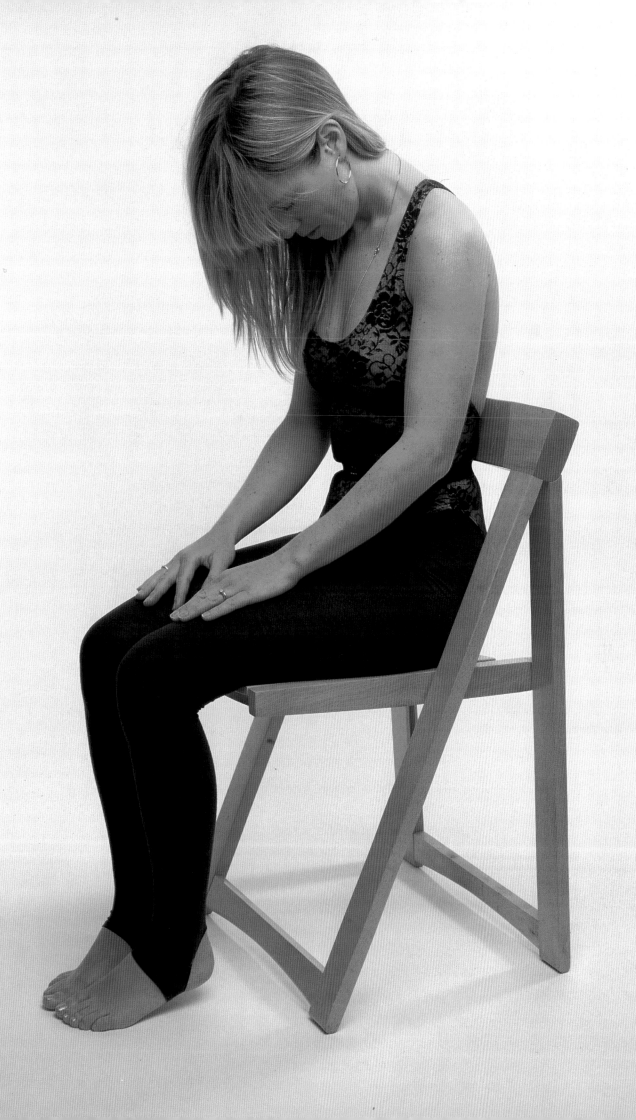

Eight Limbs of Yoga

We live by stages of evolution, which can sometimes be a slow and painful process. A sensible and well-defined way of evolving is to climb the Eight Limbs of Yoga, beginning by defining our mental and physical attitude and ending by having the ability to observe life without prejudice, simply by the act of being able to withdraw. The peace which will come with this faculty will increase courage, strength and confidence and secure a relaxed and happy outlook.

The Eight Limbs of Yoga are:

*1. **Yama**—An attitude of good conduct to others, for examples, respect for life, truthfulness, honesty, generosity, non-covetousness.*

*2. **Niyama**—an attitude of good conduct towards self, for example, cleanliness of mind and body, contentment (acceptance of life as it is, but only after having done your best to improve it), austerity (self-discipline of setting aside time for self).*

*3. **Asana**—postures. Training the body to be obedient. When the body is comfortable "opposing sensations will cease to torment".*

*4. **Pranayama**—Breath control. Breath is regulated in order to utilize Prana in the best way. Learning to calm and concentrate the mind and body.*

*5. **Pratyahara**—Sense withdrawal or relaxation. The body is under the control of the mind.*

*6. **Dharana**—Concentration. The thoughts are under control.*

*7. **Dhyana**—Meditation. Becoming one with the object on which you concentrate.*

*8. **Samadhi**—Contemplation. The will is under the control of the mind.*

Samadhi

Dhyana

Samadhi
Aristotle wrote that when human beings
rise to the level of contemplation they
achieve a glimpse of the life of God.

Dhyana, Dharana, Pratyahara
When in recollection he withdraws all his
senses from the attractions of the pleasures of
the sense, even as a tortoise withdraws all its
limbs, then his is a serene wisdom.
—*Bhagavad Gita*

Dharana

Pratyahara

Pranayama

Pranayama
All was confusion, bewildering and blind;
Unstable the heartbeat, shattered the mind.
Then came the peace; mind and body aligned.
Peace—only one Breath away.

Extend the senses, all-seeing, not blind;
Softly the heartbeat, gentle the mind.
Center, then feel mind and body aligned;
I AM—only one Breath away.
—*Juliet Shankland*

Asana

Asana
With upright body, head and neck,
which rests and move not;
with inner gaze which is not restless,
but rests still between the eyebrows.
—*Bhagavad Gita.*

Niyama

Yama

Yama and Niyama
The infinite future is before you, and you must
always remember that each word, thought and deed lays
up store for you and that as the bad thoughts and bad works
are ready to spring upon you like tigers, so also there is the
inspiring hope that the good thoughts and good deeds are
ready with the power of a hundred thousand angels to
defend you always and forever.
—*Vivekananda*

AND AFTERWARDS...

If you have attempted some Yoga you may feel you have eased out some of the knots with the stretches and felt a new clear-mindedness after Yoga breathing.

However, I hope you have become aware that there is more to Yoga than this. Yoga is about a whole day of life— about achieving your full potential spiritually. There will be a new confidence from the inner peace acquired; there will be a balanced, a less prejudiced outlook. You will dispel negativity by a positive approach to life.

Perhaps this book has encouraged you to practice Yoga with others of like mind, and at this stage I would like to sincerely thank my dear friends Kay, Shirley, June, Chrissie, Fiona, Louise, Becky and Tom for their invaluable help with it. But do bear in mind that Yoga is individual—you don't need to keep up with anyone. You will, though, I am sure, find the atmosphere when a group work together, happy, calm and serene.
Om Shanti

Peace and Love

Our deepest fear is that we are inadequate.
Our deepest fear is that we are powerful beyond measure.
It is our light, not our darkness, that most frightens us.
We ask ourselves: "Who am I to be brilliant, gorgeous, talented, fabulous?"
Actually, who are you *not* to be? You are a child of God.
Your playing small doesn't serve the world.
There's nothing enlightening about shrinking
so that other people won't feel insecure around you.
We are all meant to shine, as children do.
We were born to make manifest the glory of God that is within us.
It's not just in some of us: it's in everyone.
And as we let our own light shine,
we unconciously give other people permission to do the same.
As we're liberated from our own fear, our presence automatically liberates others.

Nelson Mandela

INDEX

PICTURE CREDITS

All pictures by **Garth Blore** except the following:

MC Picture Library: Front cover (main picture); 6; 9; 56; 122 & 123

Eugene Jones: 21 & 101